Water Retention.

Water retention and its effects on the human body.

An informative guide about water retention and its related conditions, causes, diagnosis, treatment and prevention.

by

Amelia Anderson

TABLE OF CONTENTS

INTRODUCTION

What is water retention? The simple answer is that water retention is water in the body that is in the wrong place or in the wrong amount. A person retaining water may be aware of it, such as edema surrounding a sprained ankle. Often, however, people think they've gained weight around their middle by piling on fat while it's actually water that has accumulated ... another form of water retention.

This book first describes normal water distribution in the body and the mechanisms that keep the water distributed "properly". Later chapters explore some of the many conditions in which water occurs in the wrong place and what may be done to prevent, lessen, or treat it.

Some of the conditions are rare and many need several medical specialists to diagnose and treat them. In writing this book I've been saddened by the stories of patients who've spent years first trying to find a diagnosis and then trying to treat it.

I do hope this book is useful for patients and families directly as well as pointing out useful websites for additional help. These days the wealth of information out there available to everyone is amazing.

Please note: I have used fluid instead of water throughout to indicate water that is not completely pure.

CHAPTER 1: THE BODY'S WATER

The body does a delicate dance to distribute water throughout the body. However, when things go awry, water can end up in the wrong place. The effect may be temporary and of no real concern or it may be longer lasting and pose discomfort or a health risk. To understand what goes wrong, it helps to know what happens when everything works correctly.

How much water is in the human body?

How much water there is in the body depends upon age, sex, and degree of obesity. A baby's weight is about 70% water; adult men, 60%; adult women, 50%; and obese adults, 45%.

Much of the difference in the percentage of water in various bodies is in the different amount of fat they have. Fat is only 10% water compared with bone at 20%, muscle at 75%, and blood at 92%.

Where is the body's water?

About two-thirds of the body's water is intracellular – that is, the water is inside various cells – either the cells of the body's organs (skin, muscles, heart, etc.) or individual cells such as red blood cells, white blood cells, sperm, and bacteria.

The other third of the water is "extracellular" – water that is outside of cells.

If you ask people where most of the extracellular fluid might be found they'd probably guess it's in the blood. But the fluid of blood, plasma, is not where most of the water is located. Based on the percentage of body weight, the primary extracellular fluids are:

Interstitial fluid   15%

Plasma   4%

Lymph   1%

Compartments   2-3%

Interstitial fluid is found between cells and contains nutrients being supplied to cells and waste being removed. Plasma is in the heart and blood vessels while lymph is within the lymphatic system. The compartments where water is found include the ventricles of the brain and the spinal column space, joint capsules, the eye, gastrointestinal tract, peritoneal cavity and pleural spaces.

This is where water is usually found, but individual molecules of water are not locked in place ... water is exchanged and circulated easily throughout most parts of the body, passing through capillaries and cell walls.

Normal water circulation

Normally water enters the body through food and drink. (Abnormal sources of water include medical IVs, enemas, etc. and some water is absorbed by the lungs in near drowning.) An adult normally takes in 2½ quarts of water a day: two thirds from beverages and one third from solid food and soups. A small amount of water, maybe seven ounces, is created by chemical reactions of cells within the body.

So, when we drink or eat water, where does it go? Some water is absorbed by the lining along the entire intestinal tract but most is absorbed by the villi that make up the wall of the small intestine. The water flows from capillaries in the villi to the portal vein, which brings it to the liver to be detoxified. It then travels to the right side of the heart. The heart pumps it via the pulmonary artery through the lungs. From the lungs it goes to the left side of the heart and is then pumped through the aorta to be distributed throughout the body.

The body doesn't seal water from escaping the body. We lose some through evaporation from the skin, from the lungs in respiration, through perspiration, and some is retained in the intestinal tracts and excreted with feces. About 2 quarts are excreted by the kidneys each day.

Here is an example of normal daily fluid intake and output in a 154-pound (70kg) male. Intake and output are the same and are about 84 ounces or over 2½ quarts (2.5L):

	In milliliters	In ounces
Intake		
Food	750	25
Drink	1500	51
From metabolism	250	8
Total	2500	84
Output		
Evaporation from skin and breathing	900	900
Feces	100	3
Urine	1500	51
Total	2500	84

(Source: Onur, 2015)

Very hot weather can increase water loss by as much as 7 quarts (6.6 liters) per day and strenuous exercise by at least half that. (Total body water for the 154-pound male is about 44 quarts (40 liters).

What happens when cells or the body become waterlogged or dehydrated?

If single cells or tissues dry out, capillaries usually supply additional water via the interstitial fluid. If tissues become waterlogged, water can be removed by both capillaries and the lymphatic system.

Now if the whole body becomes waterlogged or dried out, several organs are involved. The brain monitors the osmotic pressure of the blood and blood pressure. Osmotic pressure is related to the concentration of dissolved substances in a fluid. When osmotic pressure increases, the body's water content is decreasing. When osmotic pressure decreases, the body's water content is increasing. Changes in blood pressure also indicate that total fluid volume has changed – rising blood pressure is interpreted as increased fluid and dropping blood pressure as decreased fluid.

There are two primary mechanisms to keep the body's water content fairly constant: the hypothalamus and the kidney:

The hypothalamus, adrenals and the kidney

The hypothalamus is a tiny organ (the size of a pea or pearl) located on the underside of the brain. It has an area called the "thirst center" which reacts to high osmotic pressure and dry mouth to send a message to our brains that we are thirsty.

In addition to controlling thirst, the hypothalamus also, through the nearby pituitary gland, controls the adrenal glands' manufacture and release of ADH, the antidiuretic hormone. Increases in ADH opens the pores of the kidney's tubules.

- When water needs to be kept inside the body, increased ADH opens the tubule pores, allowing more water that the kidneys are filtering to return to the general circulation. The resulting urine is highly concentrated.
- If the body has enough fluid, no additional ADH is released and the pores remain closed, allowing more filtered water be excreted as dilute urine.

The adrenals and kidney without the brain

The kidneys can also control the water content of the blood without any signal from the hypothalamus. The kidneys release renin when the blood pressure in the kidney is high. Renin is an enzyme that converts a liver protein into Angiotensin II. Angiotensin II stimulates the adrenal glands to produce aldosterone, while aldosterone signals the kidneys not to excrete salt. Water is attracted to the retained salt and follows it back to general circulation.

So if the blood pressure in the kidney is low, the adrenals assume there is need to conserve water and release aldosterone.

If the blood pressure in the kidney is high, the adrenals do not release aldosterone.

Does the amount of water in the body stay constant or change day-to-day?

People who weigh themselves every day are often dismayed to find they've gained four or five pounds in one day – or delighted that they've lost four or five pounds. Daily weight fluctuations of this scale are normal. Most of these changes are from changes in the body's water content. Some is caused by people weighing themselves at different time of day, before or after urinating or having a bowel movement, and before or after strenuous exercise or exposure to heat.

Temporary weight gain from water can also result from eating a meal high in salts and sugars.

- If you eat a lot of salt in your diet, the kidney cannot excrete the excess immediately. The salt attracts water into the blood stream, increasing fluid volume and body weight.
- Carbohydrates are converted into glucose. If the body doesn't need all the glucose, it is stored as glycogen. When glycogen is stored in the muscles it causes the muscles to also take up water, and increase weight.

What happens if we just drink too little or too much water?

Drinking too little water

We know people can die from lack of water. Babies become dehydrated and die within hours if left in a hot car. An adult's refusal of food and drink is often chosen as a means of ending a life. How long it takes adults to die depends primarily upon the amount of water in the body to start with and the temperature. A healthy person deprived of food and water at a comfortable temperature may last as long as 12 days although the average is thought to be closer to 4-6 days. If in the shade but at

9

temperatures of 120°F, a previously healthy person would probably not last three days without water.

Drinking too much water

So, what if a person drinks too much water? That too can be dangerous. If a person drinks more water than his/her kidneys can handle, the blood volume increases. The increase in blood volume alone can cause problems for the heart.

The excess water in the blood dilutes the blood's sodium level, a condition called hypernatremia. In hypernatremia, the blood's sodium level becomes lower than the sodium level inside the cells. Trying to reach equilibrium, water seeps from circulation into the cells. When this happens in the brain, the brain cells swell until stopped by the skull. This causes increased pressure in the brain and may lead to seizure, coma, and potentially death.

The kidneys over a day can excrete perhaps 12.7 quarts (12 liters) of urine. So who would drink more than that? There is a form of mental illness, psychogenic polydipsia, in which patients may consume up to 21 quarts (20 liters) of water a day. Young babies are also at risk of drinking too much water if they drink several bottles of water along with over-diluted formula.

The other victims of hypernatremia or water intoxication are those who drink a large amount of water too quickly.

- A woman died in a water-drinking contest after reportedly drinking 2 gallons of water over two hours.
- Those with highly physical work in the heat and athletes like marathon runners are at risk of hypernatremia. The physical exertion leads to sweat and loss of both water and sodium. Then if the water is replaced quickly, hypernatremia results. If the water is plain water, the cause is straightforward. However, studies of Boston Marathon runners found runners to be hypernatremic at the end of the race despite drinking water with added electrolytes. A runner in the race died in 2002 from drinking too much Gatorade during the race. Researchers believe that in addition to sweating out water and salt, the

extreme athletes and laborers also have used up their cells' fuel supply. This releases ADH, which tells the kidneys to return fluid back to circulation.

- Eating contest competitors have a risky habit of drinking large amounts of water to try to stretch their stomachs, but as they haven't decreased their sodium level through exertion, their risk of hypernatremia is less than that of the extreme athletes.

CHAPTER 2: THE CAPILLARIES

There are many routes to water retention. Something can go wrong with the brain, hypothalamus, pituitary gland, adrenal gland, kidney, liver, brain, heart, skin, muscles, capillaries, or lymphatic system – just to name a few. Or several organs can "collude" to cause water retention. Often the capillaries are involved – either as a result of direct damage to them or by their reacting to chemical changes around them. It may be helpful to first know more about these tiny vessels.

The capillaries are where the arteries and veins often meet. The arteries start as large vessels, getting smaller until they are called arterioles. The arterioles then connect with the capillaries. The veins are similar, starting as large vessels, which get smaller until they are called venules. The venules then connect with capillaries. The capillaries are not straight tubes connecting the arterioles with the venules, rather capillaries form a web of tiny vessels called a capillary bed. Perhaps the most visible capillary beds are underneath our fingernails. Capillaries are just large enough to allow red blood cells to squeeze by one at a time. The capillary bed is also served by lymphatic capillaries.

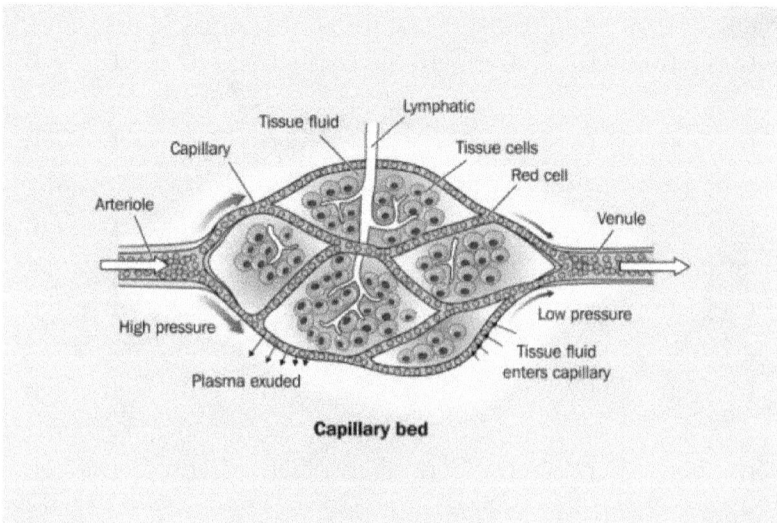

Capillary bed

There are said to be around 50,000 miles of capillaries in the human body. If all the capillaries were filled with blood at the same time, there wouldn't be any blood left for the arteries, veins or heart. What keeps this from happening? There is a band of smooth muscle called the precapillary sphincter, which can turn off the flow at the junction of the arterioles to the capillary bed and prevent blood from going through the capillary bed. The sphincter is kept closed until an elaborate system recognizes that the cells the bed serves are low on nutrients and oxygen or high on carbon dioxide and waste.

When the precapillary sphincter is closed, blood flow is diverted from arterioles directly to the venules via a vessel called an arteriovenous anastomosis.

How does the capillary bed work?
Capillaries are tubes that are only one cell thick. The cells are endothelial cells, the same kind of cells that line the larger arteries and veins.

Fat-soluble substances can pass directly through capillary walls as the endothelial cells are composed mostly of fat as well and are not a barrier to fat (it would be like water passing through a water barrier.)

The passage of other substances through the capillary walls depends on how tightly the endothelial cells are joined together. This varies by organ. Tight junctions that let nothing through are found in the brain, forming the blood brain barrier, and are at one end. At the other end are capillaries in the liver, which have large gaps (some compare them to Swiss cheese) which let plasma and big cells move in and out of blood system.

There are other systems that actively transport large molecules between capillaries, interstitial spaces, and the cells. These are interesting but not a focus of this book.

At the arteriole end of a capillary bed, the higher blood pressure forces water, ions, and nutrients into the interstitial space. Blood pressure is lower at the venule end of the capillary bed and differences in osmotic pressure attract carbon dioxide and waste products from the intracellular space into the capillaries. Which materials actually pass through the capillary depends upon the tightness of the junction between their cells.

The interstitial space is not a free-flowing watery environment. Rather it is more gel-like with collagen fibers stacked every which way. Substances pass through by diffusion (molecules and ions flowing from high to low concentrations). The space is very resistant to expansion, protecting the organs from sudden change.

Three kinds of capillaries
Capillary beds are different throughout the body. Their capillaries have been grouped depending upon their "leakiness".

Continuous capillaries

Continuous capillaries are the most common; these have tight junctions between the epithelial cells. Except in the brain, they have small clefts that allow the exchange of water, ions (sodium, chlorine), gases (oxygen and carbon dioxide), and small molecules with the intracellular space. The small molecules that are exchanged include glucose (sugar) and some hormones. White blood cells are able to squeeze through the tight junctions. The tight fit of the capillaries to the red blood cells allows them to directly transfer gases through capillary cell membranes in addition to transporting solutions.

Fenestrated capillaries

Fenestrated capillaries have tight junctions and small pores, allowing larger molecules to pass back and forth between the organ and the circulatory system. These capillaries are found in the small intestine, where they allow the absorption of nutrients in the kidneys and in many glands.

Sinusoid capillaries

These capillaries are the least common. The gaps in capillary walls are large enough to allow big cells and plasma proteins to be exchanged. Blood flows very slowly through these capillary beds. Sinusoid capillaries are found in the liver, spleen, bone marrow, and the pituitary and adrenal glands.

CHAPTER 3: WOUND HEALING: EXAMPLES OF GOOD AND BAD WATER RETENTION

Wound healing gives us a good place to start in looking at water retention in the body. Most of us have experienced swelling from cuts and bumps. What causes the swelling and is it good or bad for us?

Stages of wound healing

Whether the skin is broken or not, the basic mechanism of *successful* wound healing is similar. Scientists have identified certain steps common to most of them – it's much more complicated than most of us would ever imagine. A simplified healing process of a small wound is described below:

Stop the bleeding

- Whether the vessels damaged are large or tiny, the first action of the body is to stop it bleeding. At first, the injured vessels automatically constrict to slow loss of blood. Platelets released by the broken vessels also secrete chemicals, which strengthens the constriction.
- ATP (adenosine diphosphate) is released by cells damaged by the wound.
- ATP causes the released platelets to adhere to collagen fibers from the interstitial space and damaged cells in the wound.
- The clumped platelets attract serum thrombin. The thrombin then converts circulating fibrinogen into fibrin. Fibrin

organizes into long protein strands over the clumped platelets. Later still – another compound, an enzyme called Factor XIII, binds the fibrin strands to make stronger.
* Bleeding stops within minutes.

Inflammatory response: the inflammatory process causes redness, heat, swelling, and pain. It is not an infection, rather the reaction of the body's fight to ward off infection and clear up debris in the wound.

* Platelets release cytokines towards the end of the clot formation process. One thing that the cytokines do is increase the permeability of surrounding capillaries. This allows plasma and white blood cells to easily escape the capillaries. **This causes swelling associated within wounds – an early, beneficial form of water retention.** The swelling can also cause pain.
* Some of the cytokines also stimulate pain reaction in nerve endings.
* Platelets and injured cells also release 15 or more substances. The sequencing of the release of these chemicals is interrelated and still being studied, but somehow they manage to attract white blood cells called inflammatory cells to the wound. These are specialized white blood cells that release antibiotic chemicals to kill bacteria and enzymes to dissolve debris.
* Anti-inflammatory substances are also released towards the end of this process, which cause the eventual death of the inflammatory cells. Before they die, these cells release chemicals important in the next phase.
* The inflammatory response may last 4-5 days.

Granulation stage

* The granulation stage gets its name from its appearance when seen on a surface wound of the skin: it is covered with red or pink little bumps. The bumps are capillary buds of forming vessels.

- In this stage there is collagen being manufactured by fibroblasts to fill the wound area and the formation of new capillaries to supply energy needed for wound healing.
- The endothelial cells needed to form new capillaries are thought to come from two sources: the migration of endothelial cells from nearby vessels and "endothelial progenitors" from bone marrow. (There is an ongoing debate about the existence and characteristics of the endothelial progenitor cells). The cells are attracted to the wound from chemicals released by platelets and cells damaged by the wound when low oxygen levels occur.
- The endothelial cells multiply and attach to each other to form capillaries.
- Later in this stage specialized fibroblasts pull the wound together.
- Depending upon the location of the wound, the wound is covered with a weak collagen structure.
- This process may last just a few days or a few weeks, depending upon the severity of the wound.

Finishing stage

- The last stage involves strengthening the wound surface, and maturation of the tissue within. This stage may take weeks or years depending upon the severity of the wound.
- Most of the new blood vessels involved in healing die.
- The scar that's left is formed mostly of collagen with a few live cells and rare blood vessels. The scar is never as strong as the original tissue, about 70-80% as strong, and performs no function of the original tissue.
- Wound healing involves no cellular regeneration except in healing fetal injuries.
- Scarring is what causes problems in injuries of internal organs. For example, scars from heart attacks can lead to heart failure and/or rhythm disorders. Scars are the root of liver cirrhosis and lung fibrosis.

Where is the "bad" water retention in wound healing?

Many things can go wrong with fluid balance in wound repair.

If the initial bleeding is not stopped, or if the capillary leakage is prolonged, fluid builds up in the interstitial spaces and within tissue cells themselves. If these pressures are high enough they can cause cell death.

Sometimes cell death is caused by high interstitial fluid pressure preventing nutrients and oxygen from reaching tissue cells. Other times, high interstitial fluid pressure causes fluid volume and pressure to increase within tissue cells, upsetting normal cell metabolism.

The wound may also have damaged the lymphatic system serving the wounded area, closing an escape route for both excess cells, debris, and fluids.

Excessive cell death may cause the wound site to be larger, and delay wound healing. This delay in healing puts the wound at greater risk from infection. Sometimes, if healing is delayed too long, the wound can become chronic even without infection.

What causes increased bleeding?

Weak vessels. Many conditions cause weak walls of arteries, veins, and capillaries that don't constrict as well as healthy ones, leading to increased release of fluids at the time of the original injury. These conditions include advanced age and lack of exercise and are discussed in Chapter 4.

Low platelet count. Platelets clump with red blood cells to form a clot, the first barrier to blood leaking from an injured vessel. Platelets are tiny pieces of cells manufactured in the bone marrow and stored in the spleen. Normal platelet counts range from 150,000 to 350,000 per microliter (A microliter is a teeny amount; picture a cube with the sides the thickness of a credit card).

Blood won't clot at all if the platelet level is below 5,000 to 10,000. Levels below 50,000 can be a problem with severe wounds. Platelet counts can be too high; levels over 400,000 can cause fibrinous clots within blood vessels.

Anticoagulant drugs. These drugs include prescription drugs such as Warfarin or over the counter medicines such as aspirin and other NSAIDs.

Alcohol consumption. Drinking alcohol "thins" the blood. Moderate alcohol consumption is thought to provide some protection against intravascular clotting and heart attacks through an effect on platelets.

What causes increased capillary leakage?

Many of the chemicals released by dying cells and platelets caused the original opening of the capillaries. If cell deaths continue as a result of delayed healing, these chemicals, histamines and cytokines, keep being released, calling for an inflammatory response to continue, as well as the continuation of edema.

The injury may occur in an already damaged area, such in the legs of someone with varicose veins.

Compartment syndrome – an extreme case of increased interstitial pressure

Acute compartment syndrome is most commonly found following severe injuries to a limb such as crushing injuries and broken bones. It occurs most commonly in muscles. Muscles are arranged in compartments covered with a thick membrane called fascia. Fascia is that tough silver skin that makes some cuts of meat so tough if not removed.

Injury can cause bleeding that increases the pressure within a compartment. If the pressure gets too high it shuts off blood delivery to the muscle and nerve cells. Extreme pain follows. If not treated within hours, the cells die. A small compartment may die untreated and cause little defect. But larger compartment deaths can lead to the eventual loss of a limb.

In addition to severe injuries, compartment syndrome can occur from what appear to be minor ones; a twisted ankle, a brief squeezing injury in the workplace, someone drunk lying awkwardly. In addition, casts or bandages that are too tight can cause the syndrome.

A more chronic compartment syndrome can be caused by overdoing strenuous exercise.

Abdominal compartment syndrome can occur if abdominal fluid builds in the abdominal cavity to the point that the skin over the abdomen can't stretch any further. This puts pressure on the organs and their vasculature and can cause injury or failure of the liver, kidneys, intestines, etc.

CHAPTER 4: PERIPHERAL VASCULAR HEALTH

Peripheral vascular health is essential in keeping water in the right places. Arteries and veins need to be able to constrict if injured. The muscles of arterioles need to be strong enough to restrict blood flow through capillary beds when it isn't needed. The veins need strength to maintain valves to fight against pressure and gravity. The capillaries need to keep their cellular walls intact – either to keep their junctions tight when needed or to allow only certain sized components to flow through if this is their design.

Damage to vascular elements can lead to numerous chronic diseases and some horrible acute ones and are associated with many of the water retention conditions in the chapters that follow.

A critical component of blood vessels is the endothelium. This one-cell-deep sheet lines the inside walls of the heart, arteries, veins, and forms the capillaries. The cardiovascular endothelium is an organ the size of the liver and is said to be able to cover most of a football field. Years ago, the endothelium was considered a fairly static "hose". Later it was discovered that compounds released by the endothelium regulate blood flow and pressure, tell vessels when to dilate and constrict, regulate fluid electrolytes, control the volume of fluid inside and outside of vessels and manage coagulation. It's now thought that damaged epithelium is a direct harbinger of most cardiovascular diseases, including conditions related to water retention.

Risk Factors

Almost all risk factors for heart disease are also risk factors for endothelial disease. Most of the risk factors either directly or indirectly cause an inflammatory reaction to occur as if the vessels were attacking foreign bodies or trying to close a wound. This can end with actual destruction of endothelial cells – fragments of cells or groups of them can be found in the circulating blood of people with unhealthy endothelium.

Risk factors include:

- Age and male sex
- High cholesterol and/or Low HDL
- Diabetes
- Eating the wrong fats and sugars

- Smoking
- High blood homocysteine levels
- Obesity
- High blood pressure

Age and male sex

The cells of the endothelium can live for 30 years. When the original cells are replaced, it has been shown that the new cells are less effective, especially in producing nitrous oxide (NO). NO is produced by the endothelial cells and is important for the flexibility of the blood vessels, in its being able to relax and cause the vessels to dilate. The stiffened vessels create resistance to blood flow and make the heart work harder. NO also inhibits inflammation and the formation of thrombosis in the blood vessels. The NO is made using L-arginine, an amino acid.

The health of endothelial cells drops off gradually in men between 40 and 50 years old. In women, the cells stay healthier longer at first but then fail faster after loss of estrogen. Age is not an absolute cause of endothelial health dysfunction – it's just that the cells become less and less able to tolerate other risk factors.

Smoking

Within five minutes of exposure to cigarette smoke the endothelial cells stop producing NO. It doesn't matter if the exposure is from smoking the cigarette itself or from secondhand smoke. Research continues to discover what in the smoke is so damaging. Nicotine doesn't appear to be the primary direct culprit.

Free radicals have been implicated in smoking's danger. Free radicals are molecules with only one electron in an atom's outer orbit, making it unstable (inert compounds always have two electrons). Free radicals attack other molecules looking for weak bonds, they break the bonds, and create other free radicals. A chain reaction can follow which can kill cells. Free radicals increase with age. A healthy body's antioxidants controls free radicals, which are a common result of cellular metabolism.

Cholesterol

Cholesterol is made in the body and is essential for many purposes, including making and maintaining cell membranes, as well as being an important ingredient of steroid hormones, bile acids to digest fat, and vitamin D. It also serves to protect parts of the brain. It causes problems in the circulatory systems when it's laid down into imperfections in the endothelium.

Cholesterol is carried in the body by lipoproteins. Low-density lipoproteins (LDL) are the necessary, tiny fatty substances that transport cholesterol around the body. If LDL becomes oxidized, it deposits cholesterol in the vessels – this is why LDL is known as the bad cholesterol, although LDL isn't itself cholesterol at all.

High-density lipoproteins (HDL) vacuum any freestanding cholesterol in the body and take it back to the liver to be reprocessed. This is why the HDL is known as good cholesterol.

High blood pressure

High blood pressure causes direct endothelial damage: it decreases NO, contracts vascular smooth muscle, and causes inflammation.

Diabetes

In Type I diabetes the resulting high blood sugar is the direct cause of metabolic changes in endothelial cells.

In Type 2 diabetes, damaged endothelial cells come before diabetic symptoms.

In both forms of diabetes the damaged endothelial cells result in the poor transportation of nutrients, gases and waste through the walls. Vascular tone and flexibility is decreased, coagulation is slowed and angiogenesis is both heightened and reduced. Angiogenesis is the making of new blood vessels from existing ones. Slow defective wound healing occurs in diabetes while overgrowth of new blood vessels causes complication of the retina of the eye and of the kidneys.

Obesity

Having huge amounts of fatty tissue in the body increases the amount of substances released that are pro-inflammatory, acting directly to damage endothelium.

Eating the wrong fats and sugars

Fatty acids from partially hydrogenated vegetable oils found in oleo, pastries, and other manufactured foods are particularly harmful, causing an inflammatory reaction of endothelial cells. Studies have shown that blood vessel tone and blood flow fall shortly after a fast food breakfast high in trans fats as well as one of refined carbohydrates and sugars (Trans fats are the manufactured solid fats made from vegetable oils through hydrogenation). The deleterious effects last several hours. These effects could be prevented in a research setting with huge doses of vitamins C and E.

Increased homocysteine in the blood

High homocysteine levels are usually the result of metabolic errors in digesting proteins. It can be caused by a genetic flaw or a shortage of vitamin B and folic acid. High levels make a person more at risk for endothelial damage of blood and lymph vessels, strokes, blood clots, and heart attack.

Can the health of the endothelium be measured?

The short answer is yes. Traditionally, physicians assumed there had to be endothelial damage by assessing a person's risk factors, but they had no way to measure it directly.

For clinical diagnosis of serious cardiac disease there were invasive tests such as coronary angiography – cardiac catheterization - and cardiac Doppler. Researchers used these invasive tools to prove that endothelial dysfunction was highly correlated with cardiovascular disease. Yet they couldn't use these tools for what they really wanted to do: to diagnose early endothelial damage, predict cardiovascular disease if untreated, and monitor the success of treatment approaches.

Knowing this, researchers then began looking for less expensive and less invasive ways to measure endothelial function.

Flow mediated dilation – FMD

The first methods assessed the endothelium of large vessels such as the brachial artery, the large artery in the arm etc. A blood pressure cuff is used to cut off blood flow to the hand. After five minutes, the cuff is released and blood flows to the hand, which is crying out for oxygen. Healthy endothelium will allow the brachial artery to expand to deliver the surge of blood needed. Unhealthy endothelium has stiffened the artery and won't expand as well or may even constrict. The ability of the artery to expand is usually measured by ultrasound.

Variations of this method have used dipping a hand or foot in ice water to shut off blood supply and MRIs have been used to detected changes in an artery's response.

These methods are called FMD: flow-mediated dilatation. They are known as macro methods as they are looking at large arteries. FMD has worked well in research labs but is hard to duplicate between laboratories and in clinical settings. Research is continuing to try to standardize this approach.

Peripheral artery tonometry – PAT

The other type of method uses peripheral artery tonometry (PAT). These are micro methods that still use a blood pressure cuff to stop blood flow to the hand. But instead of measuring the size of a large artery when the pressure is released, PAT methods use tiny blood pressure cuffs on a finger to measure pressure increase in the fingertip's small arteries. There is a commercial PAT device approved by the FDA for clinical use called EndoPAT.

The EndoPAT procedure monitors the pressure in fingers of both hands. The test finger pressure is related to the control finger pressure to give a score. If the score is 1.0, it pretty much means that the peripheral arteries in the finger did not expand at all to allow increased flow, indicating serious endothelial damage. The test takes about 15 minutes.

Some studies have used EndoPAT to predict heart disease. One study of outpatients already at risk of coronary heart disease was able to used EndoPAT to predict those most at risk for future cardiovascular events such as deaths, hospitalizations, etc. (Rubinshtein, 2009)

Studies to see if various lifestyle changes or medical treatments will reduce endothelial damage have had two results: improved EndoPAT scores have been correlated with reduced cardiovascular disease in the future. Plus, if treatments are followed with no change in EndoPAT scores, it was discovered these patients are in a very high-risk group for imminent disease. (Ferré, 2010)

Many physicians find this non-invasive test useful in trying to assess patient risk for coronary heart disease. They are aware that common blood tests provide little help. For example, the data for over 100,000 patients hospitalized for acute coronary artery disease found that 77% had normal LDL, 45% normal HDL, and 61% normal triglyceride levels. (Sachdeva, 2009)

Charges for the EndoPAT test in the US are around $150/£100. Most insurers still consider the test experimental, waiting for larger studies.

Variations of PAT procedures have used infrared and temperature measurements of the fingertip.

How can endothelial damage be prevented or reversed?

Now for the really bad news. Unfortunately, the route to vascular health for most of us will be accompanied by disappointment, as it involves a healthy diet, a reasonable amount of exercise, and the avoidance of harmful habits.

Endothelial damage need not be permanent. Factors that prevent endothelial damage or reverse it include:

Not smoking	Healthy diet
Exercise	Estrogen
L-arginine	Reduced cholesterol
Lowering homocysteine	Reduced oxidized LDL

Not smoking

Smokers who stop smoking see an almost immediate drop in their blood pressure and heart rate. Studies of endothelial health using EndoPAT show improved results in endothelium eight weeks after quitting (European Society of Cardiology, 2013). Cardiovascular recovery depends quite a bit on how long a person has been smoking and how much damage is done that needs fixing. Circulation is said to improve two weeks to three months after quitting. Of course, smoking impacts many organs. Overall smoking-related deaths have been estimated to be reduced by 90% if a person stops before age 30 and by 50% if he/she stops before age 50.

Exercise

Exercise increases the production of NO, which is beneficial to endothelial health and vessel function. Studies have shown that exercise reduces inflammation of the endothelium. Exercise also increases the density of capillaries as muscles and organs call for more nutrients. With just a few weeks of inactivity, capillaries shrink. Just moving every part of the body every day helps keep these capillaries alive. Studies have shown that regular exercise, even if just stretching, can help prevent the decline in capillary function that occurs with age.

Regular to moderate aerobic exercise (it makes you breathe hard) provides the additional benefit of increased HDL lipoproteins, lessening the obstruction of the arteries. It also protects even those who are obese from oxidized LDL, which is the LDL associated with arterial disease (Kosola, 2012).

The American Heart Association calls for 150 minutes a week of moderate exercise or 75 minutes of vigorous activity. Moderate exercise is equivalent to walking 100 steps a minute; vigorous activity is usually defined as any activity that causes increased heart and breathing rates. What is vigorous depends on the underlying health of the person.

There are many sources for exercises that are right for a person's age and medical condition. A good place to start is the article on exercise in the University of Maryland Medical Center's website: http://umm.edu/health/medical/reports/articles/exercise#ixzz3JFX MfWjB.

Greater benefit from exercise is gained when combined with a decent diet.

Healthy diet

A recent review of diets and health pointed out that most of us already know what we should eat (Katz, 2014). They also noted the similarity between the many popular diets: low-carbohydrate/low fat; vegetarian and vegan; Mediterranean;

Paleolithic – they are all very similar, differing primarily in the amount of lean animal proteins. They all tell us not eat too much food, and most of it should come from plants. They all limit refined starches, added sugar, processed food, and partially hydrogenated fats.

There has been research warning that overreliance upon foods containing lectins may harm endothelial tissue. These foods include beans, grains, and tomatoes. As we've learned over the years, the best diet is one in which a wide variety of foods is consumed.

Dietary elements found to foster endothelial health:

Fiber is an often ignored but important element in the diet and aids endothelial health in a number of ways. First, it makes us feel full, reducing the urge to eat something salty, fatty, or sweet, thereby controlling or reducing the weight that results in obesity – now thought to affect half of Americans. In addition, fiber delays the breakdown of carbohydrates into sugar, preventing the blood sugar peaks that lead to diabetes. There are two types of fiber, soluble and insoluble.

Insoluble fiber helps with intestinal health and the prevention of obesity. Good sources of insoluble fiber include whole-wheat flour, wheat bran, nuts, beans and vegetables, such as cauliflower, green beans and potatoes,

Soluble fiber is soluble in water and during digestion makes a gel-like substance. Dietary sources of soluble fiber include oats, peas, beans, apples, citrus fruits, carrots, and barley.

Americans consume only about 10% of the fiber that they did 100 years ago. It is thought that a good diet should have at least 30 grams a day – about half of what most Americans consume.

Vitamin E has been shown to improve vessel tone. Dietary sources of vitamin E are a variety of vegetables, oils, meat, eggs, poultry, and cereal.

Vitamin C has improved vessel tone and counteracted effects of high levels of homocysteine. Vitamin C also improves blood flow to muscles in the elderly. Dietary sources of vitamin C include many fruits and vegetables, seafood, and animal meats – especially liver.

Antioxidants: Vitamins A and E are antioxidants. Rich dietary antioxidants are found in wine, tea, fruits, vegetables, and olive oil.

Flavonoids have been found to improve blood vessel tone. Foods high in flavonoids include dark leafy greens, dark berries (cranberries, blueberries), garlic and onions. Flavonoids are also found in dark chocolate (at least 70% cocoa), some teas, and red wine. Studies have shown that flavonoids strengthen vessel walls and valves. Flavonoid-containing foods are often recommended to relieve varicose vein symptoms.

L-arginine is an amino acid used in the body's manufacture of NO. The body usually makes an adequate supply of this compound but it has been prescribed for angina, congestive heart failure, and erectile dysfunction. Vitamin C enhances the effectiveness of L-arginine. Dietary sources of L-arginine include dairy, meat, seafood, nuts, oats, seeds, and soy.

Alpha-lipoic acid has been found in studies to be important for endothelial health. This compound is produced by the body and is found in almost all foods. Dietary sources of alpha-lipoic acid include almost all foods but are a bit higher in organ meats and green leafy vegetables.

Supplements: The use of supplements beyond those in a daily multivitamin are between you and your doctor. While vitamin C and E supplements have been found to be beneficial to endothelium, many of the studies proving it have used very high doses over short periods.

Reducing Cholesterol and Oxidized LDL

The best ways to reduce LDL and cholesterol are diet and exercise.

If medicines are needed to lower cholesterol, there are many to choose from. Yet more and more of the literature is warning of their side effects: amnesia; memory problems; increased risk of diabetes, especially in older women; neuropathies such as numbness, tingling, sensitive to touch; and muscle weakness and/or pain – the pain comes from dying muscle cells.

Statins such as Lipitor and Zocor act on the liver to reduce the body's production of cholesterol, Statins reduce the bad LDL and may cause the good HDL to increase a bit.

Niacin is a B vitamin that also lowers LDL and increases HDL. A prescription form of niacin is Niaspan.

Bile acid resins are drugs that act similarly to soluble fiber in the diet. They work in the intestine to absorb bile, allowing the bile to be excreted instead of being recycled in the liver. The liver needs to make more bile acid, using cholesterol to do so. These medicines include Questran and Welchol.

Fibrates are medicines that reduce the production of triglycerides, increasing HDL. Fibrates include Tricor and Lopid.

Combination medicines. Numerous prescription medicines now include more than one type.

Estrogen

Estrogen protects the endothelium against damage. This includes damage caused by high cholesterol and aging. At menopause, women are largely not well informed of their increased risk of cardiovascular disease. Estrogen supplement trials of post-menopausal women showed little reduction in cardiovascular disease.

Lowering homocysteine

High homocysteine levels in the blood can be caused by a genetic flaw or a shortage of vitamin B and folic acid. Alcoholics often have high levels: this is thought to be caused by both a poor diet and the direct effect of alcohol. Levels of homocysteine that aren't lowered by adequate vitamin B and folic acid consumption may be lowered by eating a diet low in methionine. Methionine is an amino acid that is not manufactured by the body. Low methionine diets avoid foods such as eggs, cheese, and fish. Lowest methionine intake is possible following a vegan diet.

CHAPTER 5: VENOUS INSUFFICIENCY AND LEG EDEMA

The previous chapter described peripheral veins and how to keep them healthy. This chapter will delve a bit into one of the more common problems with peripheral veins ... those of the legs. The veins of the legs are more affected by gravity than other veins in the body and so are usually the first to signify that your veins are not at all healthy.

The take-away message of this chapter is the importance of early diagnosis and adherence to treatment to avoid having venous insufficiency truly change your life. People too often know that vein problems run in their family and delay treatment. Even many doctors do not take diseased veins seriously, dismissing them as a wholly cosmetic, not medical, problem.

Anatomy
The leg veins carry blood from the legs back to the heart to become oxygenated. There are deep veins and superficial veins. Veins that go between the deep and superficial veins are called perforator veins. All of these veins have one-way valves which, if healthy and closed, keep blood from flowing towards the ground. The flow of blood in a healthy leg goes towards the heart, flowing from superficial to the deep veins, often via the perforator veins.

What can go wrong?
It may begin with the feeling that your legs have become heavier than usual. Your ankles swell – this not be obvious at first and is best seen when looking at the back of the leg. You may or may not already have had varicose veins or even a clot in a deeper vein. Later, first your feet and then your legs swell but you find the swelling goes away if you rest and raise your legs. Heaviness in your legs may start to be painful, itchy, or you may have restless legs at night. Later, the swelling may not go away. You have trouble standing for very long without making things worse.

The skin over your ankles may turn reddish, brown, or later black. The brown pigment is caused by red blood cells escaping the veins – their hemoglobin is broken down to brown pigment that is fairly permanent. The veins may bleed, sometimes heavily. If untreated, the skin may later turn purple and leg ulcers appear. The ulcers may be superficial at first, but they deepen. Treatment of ulcers may involve surgery on the diseased veins before they can be healed. Even when healed, ulcers often return.

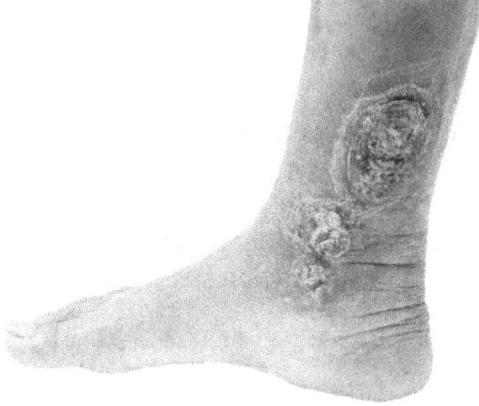

Picture: Chronic leg ulcers from venous insufficiency

What has happened?
The veins of the legs have to return blood to the heart despite the pressure of gravity upon them. It's the pressure of the foot and leg muscles upon the deep veins within muscles that pushes the blood upward. For this to happen, your feet and legs have to move. The valves of healthy veins close tight when not being squeezed so that blood doesn't flow back down.

Even when veins are healthy, if most of us stand for a long time without walking around or sitting for a while, our ankles or feet will swell a bit. Maybe the only sign of swelling is an indentation in the skin left from elastic sock tops preventing swelling at that one place.

If we don't walk enough or stand for too long, often the continued pooling of blood weakens the walls of our veins. This prevents the valves from closing tightly and blood pools more, first at the ankle but as more blood pools, the valves higher up on the leg are damaged. When valves are damaged, this is called venous insufficiency. The pooled blood reduces the supply of oxygen and nutrients to the vessels, which exacerbates the vein and surrounding damage to the skin seen in the advanced disease.

Swollen veins are described by their size, location, and associated complications in the CEAP classification system (Clinical severity; Etiology, cause; Anatomy; Pathophysiology).

- C_1 are the spider veins or telangiectasia. These are tiny (1 to 3 mm) visible dilated red or blue vessels that can be seen within the skin. They can be single vessels, a web of tiny arterioles or venule covering a large area, or involve capillary bed or beds (the size of the vessels are measured when a person is standing).
- C_2 are varicose veins. Varicose veins are larger (over 3 mm) dilated vessels under the skin.
- C_3 are varicose veins with edema.
- C_4 are conditions that have associated skin changes. The 'a' group in this category includes skin color changes and eczema. Eczema is a red, wet or dry, scaly condition varying in size. The 'b' group includes skin texture changes, a deep hardening of the tissue.
- C_5 are conditions involving a healed venous ulcer. Ulcers usually occur low in the foot, ankle, or lower leg. An ulcer is the absence of skin, which can be a tiny spot or cover large areas. They are very difficult to heal and may recur even after healing.
- C_6 are conditions involving an active venous ulcer.

Note: The website of the American College of Phlebology (www.phlebology.org) contains several good photographs of each condition from C_1 to C_6 as part of its patient information section.

One small study (3 surgeons, 78 patients, 106 legs) showed total agreement between the three doctors to be only 61% in assessing the levels. The greatest difference in opinions was in C_3 – whether edema was related to venous insufficiency and in C_4 – whether eczema was related to another cause. (Sinabulya, 2013)

How common is venous insufficiency?

If we include any of the abnormalities listed as C_1 to C_6 above, at least 80% of adults have them. Estimates of the prevalence of varicose veins are that 15% or so of men have them and 25-30% of women. Only 5% or so of people have the more advanced venous conditions, and 1% have ulcers. The conditions are less prevalent in non-industrial countries, which so far have escaped our sedentary lifestyles. In countries with established healthcare systems it's been estimated that these venous conditions require 1-2% of all healthcare costs.

What are the risk factors for serious venous disease?

- Tall people
- Obese people
- People with a history of deep vein thrombosis (clot)
- Women – the hormone progesterone weakens veins and pregnancy increases the pressure on the leg veins.
- Older people
- People with high blood pressure
- People with a family history
- People who stand in one place for long periods; retail store clerks are especially vulnerable
- People with a prior leg injury
- Smokers
- Cancer sufferers
- Chronic venous insufficiency affects about 60% known to have had a deep vein thrombosis
- Long period of required bed rest for another condition

Diagnosis

The extent of venous damage is not always apparent to the eye. An early sign is often fan-shaped veins within the skin of the edges of the foot and the ankle. Enlarged superficial veins may be obscured in obese patients or by a patients' skin thickness or color. In addition, whether the superficial veins are invisible or horribly dilated and twisted – the real problem may be just on the surface or it could be from an obstruction of the deep or perforator veins. The diagnostic issues are whether the problem is just with a weakening of surface veins that allows them to dilate under normal pressures or whether reflux is occurring. Reflux defines chronic venous insufficiency and indicates a problem with the blood travelling backwards from the deep or perforator veins towards the superficial ones and increasing venous pressure on the superficial veins.

The more commonly used diagnostic procedures in addition to a thorough history and physical exam are:

Blood pressure of the legs.

Arterial blood pressure in the legs is taken in the middle of the thigh and/or at the ankle with the patient prone or reclining less than 45 degrees. This pressure is compared to the arterial pressure taken of the arm. Depending upon the method, the leg systolic (the higher number) pressure is the same or a bit higher than in the arm. If the leg pressure is lower it can mean arterial or venous insufficiency. Other studies would be done to rule out arterial involvement, as the compression treatments used for venous insufficiency are not usually recommended when the arteries are involved.

Duplex ultrasound.

Duplex ultrasound is usually used to study any patient with veins at C_2 or higher severity. It may also be used as part of the workup for spider veins if the veins are in certain locations of the leg. This study shows the anatomy of the veins and the direction and speed of blood flow. It was first used to detect deep vein thrombosis (growing or obstructing clots) but was then found useful for the other veins. In the study, patients often stand and the ultrasound probe is traced along the vein pathways several times to take measurements.

Venogram.

Venograms used to be the gold standard for vein studies. They are still used but have been replaced as the first study is usually done by the less invasive ultrasound studies. For the venogram, radiopaque dyes are injected in the veins (usually of the foot) and a series of timed x-rays are taken to determine vein size and flow. Venograms are sometimes done with CT instead of plain x-rays. MRI studies are also performed to clarify venous anatomy.

Venograms are often the first study done when an intervention of some sort is already anticipated

Complications

For the most part, venous insufficiency isn't by itself a fatal illness, although some deaths from bleeding do occur. However, the complications are many and several are life threatening. The chronic conditions can lead to disability. In addition to pain and edema, complications include:

- **Deep vein thrombosis (DVT).** DVTs are clots in the deep veins that may cause or be caused by superficial vein problems. Superficial veins that are prone to infection (phlebitis) are also thought to be able to throw off clots to the deep veins or to the lung.
- **Pulmonary embolism.** DVTs and superficial vein clots can travel to the lungs and cause emboli, which can cause sudden death.
- **Recurrent cellulitis.** Cellulitis is a bacterial infection that spreads below the surface of the skin. Recurrent cellulitis brings a risk of necrotizing cellulitis and/or fasciitis. Necrotizing, the cause of cell death, happens when anaerobic and aerobic bacteria on the skin combine in an infection. The

anaerobes give off gases that are poorly soluble so they stay in the skin. The whole process blocks blood vessels in the skin, causing cell death and gangrene. If allowed to spread to fascia and muscle, the condition is life threatening.

- **Bone infections.** Chronic deep skin infections can spread to surrounding bone, causing the infection known as osteomyelitis. This can result in amputation.
- **Venous ulcers**. These were discussed above. Loss of skin from loss of adequate blood supply causes death of skin. If untreated, the ulcer can crater down to the bone.
- **Loss of work, disability, amputation**.
- **Secondary lymphedema**. With increased venous reflux, the blood in the vein is heading in the wrong direction. This increased the pressure on the lymphatics to transport fluid. As the veins get worse the lymphatic cells suffer the same as the cells and the thick lymphatic fluid begins to accumulate.
- **Overall decrease in quality of life**. When measured, those with C_1 and C_2 veins have the same quality of life as the general population. However, patients scoring at Levels C_3 to C_6 have quality of life scores similar to many other severe diseases such as cancer, heart failure, and COPD. (Kahn, 2004)

Prevention

Prevention or improving venous insufficiency includes any of the strategies outlined in the previous chapter: exercise, avoid obesity, and eat a healthy diet. It's important to reduce high blood pressure if it exists as this acts as an extra force against the return of blood from the legs.

Exercise: you can do targeted exercises for the ankle and calf. These exercises include standing and rising on tiptoes; sitting and pointing toes; and sitting and making circular motions with the feet. These exercises are useful for everyone during air travel or sitting for long periods.

People with either sedentary jobs or ones that require long-term standing in one place can improve vein circulation in their legs through targeted exercises, especially to build up the muscles in their lower leg. The key areas to target are ankle joint movement and calf muscle strength. Targeted exercise of these areas, plus regular exercises such as walking, swimming, bicycling, tai chi, and stretching will all help maintain the pumping action needed to keep the veins healthy.

Clothing: Wear low heeled shoes; these activate the 'vascular pump'. Avoid tight clothing at waist and groin.

For comfort, avoid heat as much as possible. Patients report having trained themselves to take cold showers for relief of their symptoms. Elevate legs when sitting or lying. Elevate the foot of the bed to help veins return blood to the heart.

Weight loss: Obesity is a risk factor for all cardiovascular diseases. For vein diseases in the legs the weight compounds the problem by having the bulk of the abdomen add pressure against the veins trying to return blood to the heart.

When possible, keep the legs at or above the level of your heart when exercising and wear a compression hose whenever exercising. Avoid weight lifting and sports that cause legs pounding on hard surfaces such as running, tennis, and racquetball. Downhill skiing restricts the movement of the ankle, affecting the ability of the muscles to pump blood to the heart; wearing the boots should be limited.

Interventions

Compression:

Compression stockings are the first line of treatment for venous insufficiency of the superficial veins. They are worn during the day and relieve symptoms of swelling, pain, and other discomforts of superficial vein conditions. They do not, however, reverse or stop the progression of venous disease.

Compression stockings are essential to wear when deep and perforator veins are affected. They are used to prevent leg ulcers from forming as well as part of the treatment if leg ulcers have already occurred. Many people don't take this prescription seriously, although it has been shown to be effective.

Progressive compression stockings are those most effective, with the compression usually highest towards the ankle. As many as half of the patients can't use these stocking as they are difficult to put on for the elderly, arthritic, or obese. They also can't be used if the skin is too fragile. Of those who begin using the stockings, as many as 30-65% stop using them – they are hot, expensive, and take some time to be effective. They should be put on when you wake up, before getting out of bed. There are many products to make putting them on easier: rubber gloves, silk liner for putting on toeless stockings, tongs, hose that zips up the back, etc. Some patients find putting them on while on the bed with the leg raised makes them easier to get on.

Compression wraps are used if the stockings cannot be. They are often a series of more than one kind of material and are applied at special clinics, by homecare nurses, or by family members or the patients themselves.

Mechanical compression devices are sometimes prescribed to patients unable to use other compression products. These devices are described in Chapter 7.

Mechanical and non-mechanical negative pressure devices. These devices are used to improve the healing of active leg ulcers. The wound is covered with a non-adherent bandage, and the area around the ulcer is sealed and linked to the pressure source. Pressure is delivered by a small battery-powered portable pump or by small vacuum canisters.

Medicines

There are no prescription medicines currently approved in the US for venous insufficiency. Plant extracts such as coumarins, flavonoids, and saponocides (horse chestnut extract) are used in Europe as venoactive substances, which act to increase the tone of veins and decrease permeability.

The oral medication pentoxifylline (Trental, Pentoxil) has shown some ability to speed up the healing of leg ulcers. The medication is prescribed primarily for peripheral artery disease.

Interventions

There are many procedures performed on veins. Medical specialists involved in vein care include dermatologists, phlebologists, interventional radiologists, and vascular or cardiac surgeons. Which specialist is involved depends on the location of the veins and the procedure needed. Interventions include:

Phlebectomy: Phlebectomy is the direct removal of a small superficial vein through a tiny skin incision.

Sclerotherapy: Sclerotherapy involves the destruction of a vein by injecting a chemical into it. Pressure is applied with a local dressing and/or compression stocking to help collapse the vein walls. The vein hardens and is absorbed, much like a bruise. Substances used for this range from concentrated salt solutions, various caustic chemicals, and foams.

Ablation: Lasers and radiofrequency (heat) are two methods used to remove larger veins. These energies are applied to the vein via a catheter. Surface lasers are sometimes used for spider veins. The long veins most often treated endovenous ablation or vein stripping are the greater and lesser saphenous veins; these are large veins but the circulation of the leg improves with these damaged veins are removed.

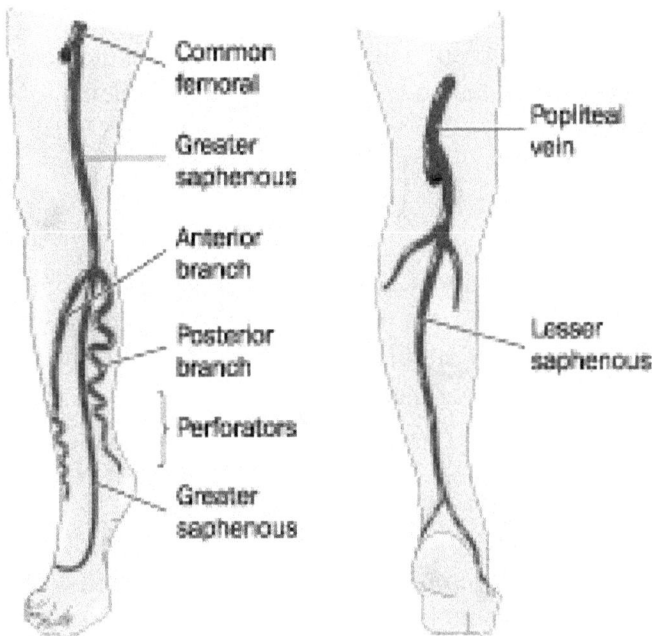

Picture: Location of greater and lesser saphenous veins at front and back of leg

Vein stripping: This is a term used when larger veins are removed through incisions in the skin. Vein stripping is done less as more physicians now use laser ablation, which has a similar success rate.

Valve repair: Sometimes the valves of large, deep veins can be repaired. This surgery is most often used to repair valves with a developmental defect.

Stent: As with stents for coronary artery disease, the vein is opened using a balloon inflated at the end of a catheter and then supporting metal mesh stents are inserted into faulty veins to keep them open. Metal stents having plastic artificial valves are currently being evaluated in animal studies. Many patents for individual artificial valves have been applied for – these would be sewn into vein walls in microsurgical procedures.

Bypass: When a section of a large vein is damaged but healthy above and below the damage, surgeons bypass the damage. Often an artificial vessel is used, such as the ones made of GORE-TEX

Reimbursement

Spider veins: The treatment of spider veins is usually considered cosmetic. Insurance does not usually cover procedures to treat spider veins unless they are bleeding or directly associated with deep vein reflux or some other issue.

Varicose veins: Treatment of varicose veins is covered with a host of caveats that vary by insurance carrier in the US. Examples of these requirements may include:
- Patient's symptoms are persistent and interfere with daily activity. Symptoms include pain, itching, swelling, cramps, or ulcer.
- Patients with multiple occurrences of phlebitis. Phlebitis is the inflammation of a vein. When this happens in a vein near the surface, there is swelling and redness of the skin. There may be a clot that has obstructed the vein, or an inflammatory reaction to cells damaged by lack of oxygen and nutrients. It is not usually an infection, although patients fear it is.
- A period of time (often 3-6 months) is often required to see if conservative treatment (compression stockings, leg elevation, exercise/reduction in sedentary lifestyle, or pain meds) will reduce the symptoms. The vein care professions have changed decisions changed in many areas for some interventions.
- Results of duplex ultrasound study or other study are required with findings consistent with the patient's symptoms. Venous insufficiency or reflux must be present in an appropriate feeder vein and that vein cannot contain a deep vein clot.

- Some surgical interventions such as vein stenting may be considered experimental or investigational. These decisions will vary by insurer.

Compression wraps: Reimbursement for compression hose and wraps is inconsistent. Some insurers cover them, the number per year varies by plan. Regular Medicare in the US covers compression hose only if needed for treating an ulcer, but many Medicare supplemental plans cover them for relieving symptoms unrelated to ulcers.

Mechanical compression devices: Some insurance companies reimburse for their use in treating leg ulcer.

Mechanical and non-mechanical negative pressure devices: Many insurance companies consider these to be investigational and not covered; other companies cover these devices after other treatments have failed.

A recent article (Schul, 2013) in Phlebology analyzed the policies of several US health insurers. They noted the lack of uniformity between insurers and the frequent modification of their rules for medical necessity within each one – which is frustrating patients and caregivers alike. Their most serious finding was that published papers considered to be important by vein experts are often ignored in policymaking. Instead, insurers seemingly picked out papers to support predetermined policies.

Support and information

The American Venous Forum (www.veinforum.org) is a professional organization open to physicians and allied health professionals who provide vein care or who are involved in vein research. AVF provides professional seminars and conferences. AVF also sponsors vein screening by members (sites are online) and also has an online venous screening scoring tool available to anyone. Among the educational materials is a 100-page book that can be downloaded free: "THE LAYMAN'S HANDBOOK OF

VENOUS DISORDERS" which is adapted from a book published by Hodder Arnold, London in 2009.

The American College of Phlebology (**www.phlebology.org**) is an organization of physicians and other health care professionals providing vein care. ACP provides professional online and offline educational programs. ACP develops standards of care, certification exams and educational materials, including an online magazine. The web site includes physician treatment guidelines for vein diseases. For patients there is an online self-assessment of veins, which include several photographs of vein disease at the C_1 to C_6 levels of severity. There is a provider locator; most providers are in the US although a few (as in one physician in the UK) are in the international file.

The National Blood Clot Alliance (www.stoptheclot.org) is an organization established by patients and medical professionals (who were also patients). It provides several online courses giving continuing education credits for physicians, nurses, and many other health professionals. It also has a wide array of information for patients, including those concerned with deep vein clots, which often are the cause of venous insufficiency.

Varistop.com is a support group that includes product reviews written by patients and a blog with discussions of compression products. The site has a good section on how to exercise safely.

The Circulation Foundation (www.circulationfoundation.org.uk.) is a UK group founded by vascular surgeons and is open to physicians and other health care professionals providing vein care. The foundation finances research and has online patient education materials including a risk checker.

Chronic Venous Insufficiency Network is a small closed group on Facebook.

Many large medical centers have excellent educational materials online, as do other professional vein care professional groups.

There are also many different physician specialties that care for people with vein problems – many of these provide patient information on their websites.

Patient out-of-pocket costs

In the US, treatment of spider veins will usually be paid for by the patients as will some vein treatments. The cost of treatment depends on the size of the area to be treated. Sclerotherapy and superficial laser treatments run at $200-500 (£130-335) per treatment and as many as six or more treatments may be required. Endovenous treatments range from $1,500-4,000 (£1,005-2,680). Surgical vein stripping (which is usually covered by insurance) may cost $10,000 (£6,700) or more (hospital direct costs for vein stripping may be $6,000 and endovenous ablation with laser or microwave, $5,000 (£3,350); what they charge to patients is always greater to cover bad debts and other indirect costs).

Compression hose and other garments depend upon the quality of the hose and the strength of the compression needed. Usually if insurance covers some of the cost it will be for the stronger progressive compression hose of at least 20mm Hg pressure. Recent years has brought more products and lower costs of many. While full price of the hose may be quoted as $30-100 (£20-67), usually online options can be found at half that amount.

CHAPTER 6: WOMEN AND WATER

Both sexes are prone to various conditions that can cause water retention, but only women can be affected by menstrual cycles, pregnancy, or menopause.

Menstrual cycle abc's

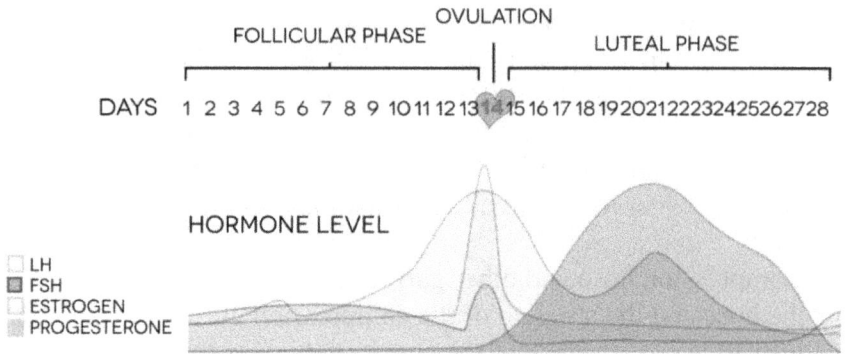

Picture: Major hormones of the menstrual cycle

There are four major hormones involved in regulating a woman's menstrual cycle. The choice of Day 1 to begin the cycle was made as it's the only time in the cycle a woman can pinpoint accurately: the beginning of the menstrual period or flow. The lining of the uterus thickens just in case a fertilized egg is released; when that doesn't happen the extra cells are sloughed off, a period that takes an average of five days and ranges from three to seven days. The entire cycle is usually described to be 28 days but cycles may vary by a week either way.

Menstrual cycle without egg being fertilized

At the beginning of the cycle, the blood levels of the hormones produced by the ovaries are low – estrogen is low and progesterone extremely low. The brain detects the low levels and signals the pituitary gland to release FSH. FSH, or follicle stimulating hormone, causes several immature eggs to begin to mature. Usually one of the eggs matures faster and begins to produce hormones of its own. The first hormones the egg releases are thought to stop the other eggs from developing. Fraternal twins are the result of two eggs maturing in the same cycle.

When the mature egg is close to ready it releases an increasing amount of estrogen. The high estrogen level stimulates the pituitary gland to release LH, the luteinizing hormone, which triggers changes in the mature egg resulting in its release.

After the egg is released, the egg's capsule becomes the corpus luteum, which produces both estrogen and progesterone. The high levels of estrogen and progesterone cause the uterus to thicken and also suppress the pituitary from releasing FSH, preventing any new eggs from maturing during the cycle.

Eventually the corpus luteum breaks apart, levels of estrogen and progesterone fall, menstrual flow ensues, the pituitary starts secreting FSH again and a new cycle begins.

Premenstrual water retention

Most women have some edema related to their menstrual cycle. This type of edema is usually generalized and peaks during the last half of the cycle, which is called the premenstrual time. Swelling of the breasts, legs, and abdomen are common complaints of women. As many as 40-60% of women experience this, though it's a serious complaint for 15% or less. It's not unusual for these more affected women to gain and lose as much as 10 pounds of water during their cycles. Both estrogen and progesterone can cause capillaries to leak fluid into the interstitial spaces and may be the source of more moderate symptoms.

PMS-H

In the past all symptoms women experienced during a menstrual cycle were lumped together for research and medical treatment.

Premenstrual syndrome (PMS) was the name given to the 150 or so possible symptoms ranging from emotional (anxiety, depression), behavioral (aggression) and physical (acne, pain, water retention, GI problems). PMS has since been divided into several subgroups. Of interest for this book is Subgroup H. The "H" stands for heaviness.

PMS-H women gain at least three pounds each month, have abdominal bloating, abnormal breast swelling, and swelling of face, hands, and ankles. The swelling for this group is mostly in interstitial spaces. The culprit is currently thought to be an excess of aldosterone.

Aldosterone

Aldosterone is a renal hormone and acts upon the kidney, causing it to retain both salt and water. Progesterone is a very similar chemically to aldosterone and is thought to mimic its action somewhat, and may contribute to edema.

One early study compared women with several severe physical PMS symptoms and women with few and less serious symptoms. All in the PMS group had fluid retention symptoms. The two groups had similar estrogen and progesterone levels, but the PMS women had much higher aldosterone levels during the latter part of their menstrual cycle, coinciding with the timing of their fluid symptoms.

The two groups were tested several times for plasma volume changes when they went from lying down to standing up. During all but the latter part of their cycles, the results of the two groups were the same: their plasma volume increased upon standing – this is from the pull of gravity filling vessels in the lower part of the body. The additional fluid comes from interstitial spaces.

Where the two groups differed was during the latter part of their cycles. Women without severe PMS had the same increase in plasma volume as other times, but the PMS group had no increase at all. This despite the PMS group having more interstitial fluid than at any other time – as evidenced by their multiple water retention symptoms. It is thought that the fluid in the interstitial spaces of this group is locked in, probably as a result of its higher salt and albumin content.

What could cause the high aldosterone levels?

- Estrogen –High levels of estrogen or the way it's broken down in the liver may cause increased production of angiotensin II. This hormone is part of the renin-angiotensin-aldosterone system, which regulates long-term blood pressure and interstitial fluid volume.

- Stress – With stress, the pituitary gland increases ACTH, which acts on adrenal gland to increase aldosterone.

- Dopamine deficiency – dopamine normally keeps aldosterone under control; dopamine also acts as a diuretic, reducing extracellular fluid.

- High serotonin levels – some have reported high serotonin levels with PMS-H. For most forms of PMS, *low* serotonin levels are associated with the behavioral and emotional symptoms. High serotonin levels, whatever their cause, will act like stress upon the pituitary and adrenal glands.

- High angiotensin II levels: some patients with high blood pressure have high angiotensin II levels, which can increase aldosterone.

- Diet – among other thing, too much refined sugar stimulates the adrenal glands, increasing the release of aldosterone.

Other causes of premenstrual water retention

- Some swelling of the breasts is normal and is mostly a response to hormones preparing the breast for breastfeeding. During the first half of the cycle estrogen causes development of the breast ducts. During the second half of the cycle, progesterone promotes enlargement of milk glands and edema, causing the swelling and tenderness often felt by women.

- Studies have shown that obesity is much higher in PMS women – and obesity is by itself a risk factor for water retention. A number of studies show women crave carbohydrates towards the end of their cycle; much of this a reaction to low serotonin levels and this can lead to weight gain which is additive rather than cyclic.

How can premenstrual water retention be lessened or prevented?

Exercise

Fat cells produce estrogen. Exercise can burn fat cells if of the right intensity and length. Running around the block for 10-15 minutes burns carbohydrates and leaves fat alone. Longer, steadier moderate exercise equivalent to 100 steps a minute will result in some fat loss and some lowering of estrogen. So do that walk or your favorite exercise for a half hour or more.

Fat cells also produce leptin, another hormone. Leptin reacts with the brain to control appetite. Overweight people may have leptin levels that are so high that the brain can't interpret it and doesn't turn appetite signals off.

Any weight reduction from exercise will also reduce or prevent obesity, a risk factor for water retention.

Exercise has been shown to reduce stress and anxiety. Study results vary but point towards the benefit of regular aerobic exercise (you can't talk comfortably during these) of 25 minutes or so. Stress can also be reduce through less aerobic practices of yoga or tai-chi. Meditation is also effective.

Medicines, herbs, etc.

Antidepressants

Antidepressants containing sertraline (such as Zoloft) have been found effective in reducing water retention related to PMS-H. These are often given just during the last two weeks of the cycle.

These drugs are believed to prevent serotonin to be recycled, reducing the amount in the body. As with any drug these medicines may have serious side effects.

Hormone Therapy

Depending upon the level of estrogen, physicians may prescribe hormone therapy.

Chrysin

Chrysin is mentioned here as something to avoid. Some articles on the Internet and some producers of supplements market chrysin as an estrogen blocker. Chrysin is found in some foods (celery, broccoli, honey). In laboratory studies chrysin has been found to inhibit aromatase only in test tubes and Petrie dishes. Aromatase is a building block for estrogen in both men and women. The supplement is purchased mostly by men to help in body building in an attempt to decrease estrogen. Despite the claims, studies have shown the chrysin is metabolized in the body almost immediately and is not available to cells.

Diet

A few details are shown below, but the basic message is to follow a healthy diet as discussed in Chapter 4.

- For lowering estrogen peaks: high fiber vegetables, low dairy, low or no alcohol, avoid sugar.
- For increasing dopamine: avoid soy, have regular small amounts of protein for every meal.
- General PMS-H measures: avoid salt, caffeine, teas, chocolate, cola, yerba mate, and guarana.
- Supplements: A daily multivitamin with adequate calcium and magnesium. Licorice root has been suggested by some, but as it can mimic estrogen it doesn't seem to make sense. Licorice root also has many serious side effects: see MedlinePlus, the website of the National Institutes of Health to check out any drug or supplements.

Menopause and water retention

Menopause is a bit like Day 1 of the menstrual cycle in that it's an exact date – the date of the last menstrual period. The date may not be known if menopause occurred naturally as a woman's menstrual periods may come and go – and the last one only vaguely remembered. Periods are skipped, as many cycles don't have a mature egg or corpus luteum, so the uterine wall doesn't thicken.

Surgical menopause occurs if a woman's ovaries are removed, with or without removal of the uterus.

Perimenopause is the word used to describe the time before menopause when hormone levels begin to fluctuate and cause symptoms. Women differ greatly in the age the symptoms begin – anywhere from the mid 30's to late 40's for most. Symptoms can last any time from 2-3 years to 12-25 years. The number of symptoms are legion but a few of the more commonly mentioned are shown below. Water retention occurs but is usually not one of the prime complaints.

- Hot and cold flushes
- Mood swings
- Weight gain
- Heightened PMS symptoms
- Irregular periods – shorter, longer, lighter or heavier flow
- Gastrointestinal symptoms from nausea, indigestion, gas, pain, bloating
- Sex – pain, disinterest
- Urinary symptoms
- Tired, trouble sleeping

What's happening with the hormones during perimenopause?

Female fetuses have 6-7 million egg follicles and one or two million remain at birth. By puberty, girls have 300,000 to 400,000 follicles, which fall to 10,000 to 30,000 by their late 30s. By perimenopause, women have a depleted supply of follicles; those that remain are less responsive to FSH and LH, thus producing less estrogen. Fewer follicles develop into a mature egg so there are fewer cycles with a corpus luteum to secrete progesterone. These lower hormone levels signal the pituitary to release higher and higher levels of FSH and LH, in an attempt to stimulate the follicles. Many of the common symptoms of perimenopause (hot flushes, forgetfulness, vaginal dryness) are a reaction to the high FSH levels. Reported sleep problems don't seem related to hormone levels.

During this time the levels of active testosterone in the body are decreasing just a bit – as long as the number of fat cells in the body remain the same. Testosterone is secreted in small amounts by the ovaries and the adrenal gland before menopause. After menopause, it is still secreted by the adrenal gland but it is also being created in fat cells, which make it from androstenedione, a precursor of both estrogen and testosterone.

What causes water retention and bloating during perimenopause?

Water retention: While estrogen levels are falling they can have peaks that are much, much higher during perimenopause than at any other time in a woman's life. This is a result of the FSH pushing the ovaries to develop follicles. Estrogen by itself can cause capillaries to leak and cause water retention. While hormone replacement therapy (HRT) is often prescribed for severe emotional and hot flush symptoms, they also rein in the pituitary and lower FSH levels.

Estrogen plus progestin is given if the uterus is intact; estrogen alone if not. HRT doses are as low as possible and given for as short a time as possible to avoid serious complications such as strokes and blood clots.

Usually progesterone counteracts estrogen's effect on water retention. As progesterone is decreasing during perimenopause, the body is more sensitive to estrogen, increasing water retention.

Some women experience water retention from HRT if prescribed during this time; this has the same causes as premenstrual water retention.

GI symptoms: Often the reported bloating symptoms during menopause are sensations from the gastrointestinal tract. Low hormone levels, especially low estrogen, which occur during perimenopause, are thought to influence the speed of digestion (both increase and decrease) and cause many of the symptoms expressed by women.

In addition, estrogen and cortisol work to balance each other. As estrogen decreases, cortisol's effect can increase stress on the body, which can affect digestive speed. This is demonstrated by studies of women who already have stress-related problems such gastric reflux disease or irritable bowel syndrome: they have more severe symptoms during their regular menstrual cycle when estrogen and progesterone levels are lowest.

Some GI problems reported by women have been found to be a temporary result of their change to a healthy diet with more fiber, fruit, and vegetables. Other problems reported as perimenopausal are simply the result of aging.

Beyond HRT, health diet, exercise, and drinking plenty of water are often recommended to reduce GI symptoms. HRT has no effect.

After menopause, is there still estrogen and testosterone in the body?

Estrogen is really a group of hormones, primarily **estriol**, produced by the placenta during pregnancy; **estradiol**, produced by developing follicles in the ovary; and **estrone**, produced by the ovary and fat cells throughout the body.

At menopause, there is no more production of estriol or estradiol. Estrone, however, continues to be produced by fat cells, the liver and muscle. This is the weaker form of estrogen also found in men. It uses the same precursor, androstenedione, as for testosterone. Before menopause, about half of androstenedione is produced by the ovaries and half by the adrenal glands. After menopause, it is still being produced by the adrenal glands.

Visceral fat cells become important in menopause as they contain large amounts of aromatase, a building block for androstenedione. The more visceral fat cells (fat not under the skin but within the abdominal cavity) you have, the higher the testosterone and estrone levels will be. Testosterone is highly correlated with production of more visceral fat.

It's a vicious cycle … the more belly fat you have the more you'll get! Getting back to the causes of endothelial dysfunction, which can lead to local or generalized water retention and the stiffening the lining of the entire cardiovascular system, an important risk factor is obesity. So increasing belly fat in menopausal women can have serious cardiovascular outcomes as well as edema.

Note: just a few numbers about fat cells. A normal adult has perhaps 25-30 billion fat cells. And overweight person has 75 billion fat cells while an obese person can have *250-300 billion of them*.

Water retention in pregnancy

There are two types of water retention in pregnancy: pregnancy edema and eclampsia.

Pregnancy edema
In pregnancy edema, swelling of the legs and feet are the most common symptoms and are experienced by at least 80% of women. The swelling gets worse as the day goes on but recedes during the night. It is most common in the last three or four months of the pregnancy. Symptoms usually disappear shortly after birth. Women are cautioned to have these symptoms monitored by their healthcare provider.

What causes pregnancy edema?

First of all, there is more fluid for the body to process. Pregnancy causes blood volume to increase 30-50% to support the needs of the growing fetus and uterine structure. Early in the pregnancy, progesterone causes the blood vessels to relax, decreasing their resistance to flow by 20% or so. This helps the body to accommodate the new fluids without increasing blood pressure. It also may cause lightheadedness early on.

The blood itself also changes: while the total blood volume increases 30-50%, red blood cells in the blood increase by only 20-30%. There is also less protein in the blood. As the blood has less "stuff" in it, it has lower osmotic pressure to suck back any fluids leaking into interstitial spaces.

As the pregnancy reaches the final months, the uterus presses against the major veins, impeding fluid from escaping the lower part of the body. This pressure also hinders the lymphatic system's escape route for fluid. Fluids from the arteries continue to reach the uterus, causing more and more fluid to leak into the interstitial spaces. There is also an increase in hormones such as aldosterone, which encourage the kidneys not to excrete sodium. Aldosterone has been mentioned earlier as the probable culprit in causing water retention in the premenstrual syndrome heaviness group.

Can pregnancy edema be prevented or lessened?

- The inferior vena cava is a large vein that allows blood from the lower extremities to return to the heart. This vein runs behind the abdominal organs along the right side of the spinal column. To relieve pressure from the uterus on the vein and allow fluid to leave the lower extremities, women are warned to avoid sleeping on their back and to favor lying on their left side.
- Drink plenty of water. This prevents the body from trying to retain both salt and water.

- Don't stay in one position very long. Get up, but don't stand in one place for more than 10-20 minutes. Move about. Stretch. Take walks. Try water aerobics.
- When sitting, keep your feet up. If the legs are swollen, apply cool compresses 10-15 minutes at a time.
- Eat a healthy diet – lay off the salt. Get enough potassium. Watch the caffeine.
- Keep cool.
- Wear loose clothing. Have shoes that have room for your feet at the end of the day. Avoid any tight bands of socks at the ankle or above the calf.
- Invest in good pregnancy compression tights. Put them on as soon as you get out of bed in the morning.

Are there any danger signs to watch for?

- If one leg is swelling more than the other it may signify a blot clot in a deep vein. During the latter part of the pregnancy the blood is hypercoagulated. This is a natural mechanism to avoid major blood loss during birth but it does increase the risk of a clot blocking a vein.
- Any sudden worsening of symptoms. It is rare but there can be medical emergencies involving swelling.
- Any symptoms that suggest pre-eclampsia, which is discussed below.

Can pregnancy cause varicose veins in addition to leg swelling?

Yes. The hormones that ready the body for pregnancy relax both the veins and the supporting tissue. The valves separate somewhat and aren't tight enough to prevent backflow, especially as the pressure from the heavier uterus during the last months of pregnancy. So the veins bulge from the added volume and become visible. As many as 40% of women have these varicose veins during pregnancy.

If the woman did not have varicose veins before pregnancy, most will see them disappear within a year after they deliver. In subsequent pregnancies women report having varicose veins earlier and larger each time.

Pregnancy is one of the risk factors for permanent varicose veins, and risks increase a little with each birth. But there are many other risk factors including heredity, diet, having a job that requires standing, and general lifestyle. Communities in the so-called third world with plenty of fiber in their diets and which lack a sedentary lifestyle have almost no incidence at all of varicose veins.

Pre-eclampsia and eclampsia

Pre-eclampsia and eclampsia are conditions that begin with problems in attaching the placenta to the uterus. Arteries don't form properly, restricting blood flow to the placenta and fetus. The lack of oxygen that follows starts an inflammatory process causing body-wide endothelial dysfunction if allowed to progress. Often the first sign of trouble is water retention beyond that experienced in normal pregnancy. Pre-eclampsia and eclampsia can cause both maternal and fetal death.

Signs of pre-eclampsia:

- **High blood pressure** in a woman who had normal pressure before. This is caused by constriction of blood vessels throughout the body from endothelial dysfunction. High blood pressure is anything above 140/90 mm.
- **Extreme and/or sudden** swelling that includes not only the lower extremities but also the hands and face. This is a result of capillaries leaking protein and fluids into the interstitial spaces and of the high blood pressure. One symptom of overall fluid retention is a weight gain of two or more pounds in a single week.
- **Protein in the urine.** Capillaries are leaking all over the body. When this happens in the kidney, protein leaks into the urine.

- **Poor development of the fetus.** The attachment difficulty of the placenta to the uterus may slow the growth of the fetus. Also, absence of normal amniotic fluid may be seen.

Possible signs of severe pre-eclampsia

- **Headache** is a symptom that is followed closely as it may signal an imminent seizure. Other neurological signs include dizziness.
- **Reflexes are brisk, over reactive**
- **Blood pressure** increases to 160/100 mm or higher
- **Protein in urine** increases
- **Vision changes** – can be blurry vision, sensitivity to light, double vision, or partial loss of vision.
- **Abdominal pain**, right upper quadrant (can be sign that liver is swelling)
- **Rapid weight gain** over one or two days
- **Decreased urine output**
- **Fluid in lungs**

What is eclampsia?

Eclampsia is usually defined as having an unexplained grand mal seizure or coma during pregnancy following symptoms of pre-eclampsia. It occurs when pre-eclampsia is not treated and the constricted vessels caused a lack of oxygen to the brain. Most often patients progress from mild to severe pre-eclampsia and then to eclampsia but some women (about 25%) progress from a relatively mild pre-eclampsia directly to seizures.

When during a pregnancy can this occur?

Pre-eclampsia can occur any time after 20 weeks of pregnancy, but usually occurs later. About 90% of the time it happens after the 34th week, and 5% after birth.

Almost all instances of eclampsia occur before delivery: 25% before labor and 50% during labor. Another 25% of cases occur after delivery.

Are these conditions common?

Statistics vary but about 5% of all US and UK pregnancies are thought to involve pre-eclampsia to some degree. The incidence among healthy women having their first pregnancy the incidence is between 2-6%.

What are the risk factors for pre-eclampsia or eclampsia?

Those at highest risk are those who've had pre-eclampsia or eclampsia before or have a family history (both mother and father) of these conditions. Also at risk are those that have experienced poor birth outcomes in the past.

Other risk factors are numerous and include:

- Having first child
- Age – teenager or over 40
- Chronic high blood pressure
- Low economic status
- History of diabetes or having pregnancy-related diabetes
- History kidney condition
- Obesity
- Having multiple births
- Having an autoimmune disease
- Having one of the thrombophilias – problem with blood clots forming too easily

Can pre-eclampsia and eclampsia be prevented?

- Studies have shown a possible reduction in pre-eclampsia when high-risk mothers are given low dose aspirin once a day if started early in the pregnancy.

- There also have been studies of L-arginine as a preventative. As described earlier in the book, L-arginine is an amino acid used to make manufacture nitrous oxide (NO), which relaxes the blood vessels. Dietary supplements of L-arginine have been shown in studies to reduce pre-eclampsia by as much as 50%. Dietary sources of L-arginine include dairy, meat, seafood, nuts, oats, seeds, and soy. Vitamin C enhances the effectiveness of L-arginine.
- Eclampsia can be prevented by picking up on early symptoms of pre-eclampsia and treating them. This is a solid case for adhering to scheduled prenatal visits.
- Early in the pregnancy, any risk factors that can be controlled are targeted.

What are the treatments?

The only effective treatment for pre-eclampsia and eclampsia is the birth of the baby.

If pregnancy is at 36-37 weeks, delivery is performed for even mild pre-eclampsia. If pre-eclampsia is severe, birth is attempted as early as 24 weeks.

For pregnancies between 24 and 36 weeks accompanied with mild pre-eclampsia, the woman and fetus are monitored closely and symptoms treated as long as it is considered safe.

Advances in diagnosis

There are now screening protocols and screening diagnostic blood tests. Studies have shown that the relation of two serum components is a good predictor of pre-eclampsia and its potential seriousness. The two are PGF, placental growth hormone and sfit-1, a tyrosine kinase protein. PGF is needed for placental growth and sfit-1 reduces available PGF. Assays for these compounds are now available in a fast, fairly inexpensive kit form.

What are the outcomes?

Maternal and fetal deaths: Maternal perinatal deaths from eclampsia in the US and UK is 6-12%. Perinatal deaths are those that are ascribed to eclampsia but which could occur up to one year after delivery.

Reported fetal deaths from eclampsia range from 13-30%.

Maternal death rates at time of delivery from eclampsia are 6.4 deaths/10,000 total births (0.6%) in the U.S.

Other outcomes: Women can suffer permanent brain damage from prolonged seizures, causing lack of oxygen to the brain. Long-term studies of women show a population with higher incidence of chronic high blood pressure, diabetes and many chronic conditions including those of the heart, kidney, thyroid, and brain. Women have higher death rates from cardiovascular causes. Studies continue to delve into how much of this is a result of just the pre-eclampsia itself or if these were predisposing conditions that led pre-eclampsia.

The long-term effects of eclampsia on the babies that survive are primarily those related to pre-term births.

CHAPTER 7: SWELLING RISING FROM THE LYMPHATIC SYSTEM

Most of us are seldom aware that we even have a lymphatic system. Our kids may have had swollen tonsils, or we may have had a swollen lymph gland or two, but this system is critical for fighting diseases, digesting fat, and removing cell waste and pathogens from the body. When the lymph system goes haywire, it can create massive damage to the body.

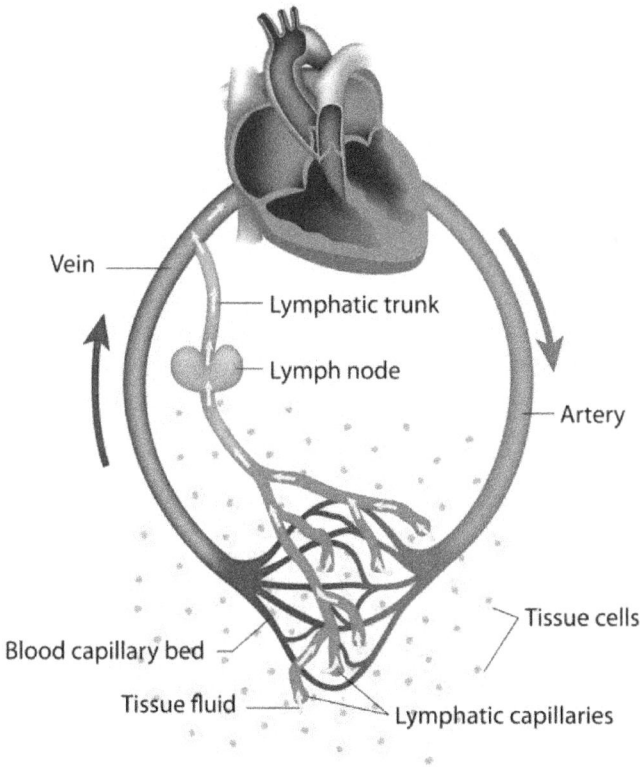

Picture: Lymphatic Circulation

Lymph circulates through the body but does it quietly – no beating heart.

The lymphatic circulatory system goes just one-way — from the spaces between the body's cells (the extracellular space) to the neck veins in the cardiovascular system. The lymphatic circulatory system serves three major functions:

1. Removing cell waste

The lymphatic capillaries remove large proteins and associated water from extracellular spaces. The fluid, called lymph, travels to veins in the neck via larger and larger vessels resembling veins. The proteins are those that are too large to be absorbed in the venous end of the capillary beds and include waste of all sort including bacteria, viruses, cell fragments, toxins, and cancer cells. Unfortunately, the lymph circulatory system also serves to spread cancer cells. Indeed, some cancers are felt to have the ability to stimulate the lymph system to do so.

2. Infection control

On the way to the neck, lymph passes through several lymph nodes. The lymph nodes are fibrous organs filled with stored white blood cells and are well connected to the blood supply. This is where the lymph's cellular waste is handed off to veins. There are 500-600 lymph nodes in the body.

White blood cells attack and destroy pathogens in the node itself as well as trigger body-wide immune responses. The nodes are sites for antibody production. During an infection, white blood cells multiply in the nodes and are released aimed at specific targets. The nodes become swollen when the nodes are producing antibodies and white blood cells to fight an invading organism.

3. Digestion

Special lymph capillaries called lacteals are in the lining of the intestinal tract. The lacteals absorb fats and water-soluble vitamins from the small intestine and add them to the flow of lymph to the neck vein.

Structure of lymph circulatory system

Lymph capillaries are a single cell thick, just like the capillaries of the blood system. The capillaries are formed from venous epithelial cells during fetal growth. The capillary structure is of loose overlapping cells that collapse when extracellular pressure is low and open when it builds up. The capillaries are intertwined with arterioles and venules in capillary beds throughout the body. Only the central nervous system, bone marrow, bones, teeth, and the cornea of the eye are not within the lymph system.

The lymph capillaries enter into larger vessels, which are similar to veins, having closely spaced valves to prevent backflow. The larger of the vessels are called trunks and these lead to veins in the neck to deliver lymph to the heart. The system is not symmetrical. The right trunk drains the right arm and the right side from the head to just above the waist. The left trunk drains the rest of the body, including both legs.

Lymph is propelled towards the heart by movements of skeletal muscles and organs upon all the lymph vessels and contraction of muscle walls of the larger lymph vessels. In addition to its circulatory system, other parts of the lymphatic/immune system include:

Organ	What it does
Red bone marrow	Produces white blood cells
Spleen	Acts much like a large lymph node except it filters waste from blood instead of lymph.
	Has similar role in infection control to lymph nodes
Thymus	Matures T-cells – a special type of white blood cell which attacks a specific antigen.
Tonsils/adenoids	Collect and destroy organisms entering the mouth.

Site of some T-cell maturation

Peyer's patches   Survey antigens in the intestine and begin immune
                           response to pathogens

When the lymphatic system goes wrong

The edema from lymphatic system breakdown is different from
blood system edema in that the lymph is a high protein fluid.
When the lymphatic capillaries are blocked, the high protein fluid
accumulates in the extracellular space – it has nowhere to go. This
fluid attracts water from the vascular system increasing the
edema, putting more pressure on surrounding cells and vessels
and damaging them.

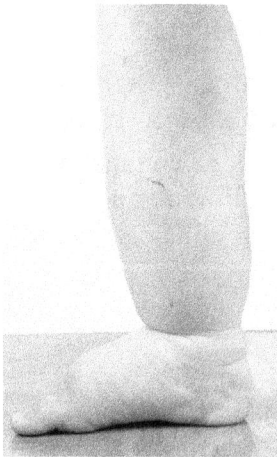

Picture: Lymphedema of leg & foot

Causes of lymphedema are grouped into primary and secondary
causes. Regardless of the cause, the treatments are similar, as are
the complications of not diagnosing it early.

Primary lymphedemas are inherited conditions that are very rare,
occurring in about one per 6,000 to 10,000 persons. Females are
affected three times more than males. The lymphatic
malformation is present at birth but may not be apparent until age

35. Usually it is the lower limb that's affected. There are three types of malformation:

- Hypoplastic. These are the most common, consisting of smaller and fewer vessels and nodes.
- Hyperplastic. Enlargement of the vessel diameter causes many of the valves to fail over time.
- Aplastic. No lymph nodes or no vessels or neither node nor vessel is present in an area of the body.

Secondary lymphedemas are caused by something blocking the lymph vessels. The causes are many, but in the United States this occurs most often as a complication of surgery, especially of breast cancer with radiation treatment and/or removal of the lymph nodes in the armpit.

In many parts of the world the primary cause is from filariasis, an infection from several species of nematode (worm) carried by mosquitos. The worm matures in the lymph system, with each mature female releasing millions of offspring. Many years may pass before the infection is known, often after the lymph system is seriously damaged. Most affected are the legs, maybe 80%. The rms, face, genitals, and the torso are also affected. An estimated 120 million people worldwide are infected by the worm, with about 40 million being severely disfigured by the disease, which is also known as elephantiasis. This condition is commonly found in poor and rural areas of Africa, Egypt, Asia, and the Pacific Islands. In the Americas, the condition is found in Haiti, the Dominican Republic, Guyana, and Brazil. In the US, the last outbreak in South Carolina died out in the early 1900s. Short visits by tourists to areas where the worm is endemic do not seem to be affected. Cases of lymphedema caused by the worm and diagnosed in the US and UK are usually in immigrant populations.

Other causes/risks of secondary lymphedema include:

- Morbid obesity, or having a body weight that is more than the frame can support. It's often said to be 100 pounds over an ideal body weight or a BMI of 40 or higher. Includes about 3% of Americans.

- Lymphangitis. This is when a localized infection enters and attacks the lymph channels; this can be hidden or obvious as when a superficial wound on the skin develops the red streaks that travel up a limb.
- Cellulitis. Deep infections of the skin. Especially if cellulitis occurs repeatedly in the same area.
- Trauma. Deep bruising and burns.
- Any surgery, including those for varicose veins or circumcision. Risk increases with radiation treatment.
- Obstruction by malignancy.
- Untreated venous insufficiency or from deep vein thrombosis (clot).
- Lipedema. This is a disease of women. It involves progressive increase in fat tissue that is unrelated to body size or obesity. It usually involves the legs, and doesn't affect the feet. Arms are sometimes involved. Lymphedema is a frequent complication.

Prevention

Lymph vessels are lined with endothelium, the same cells that line the cardiovascular system. Any of the guidelines to maintain endothelial health in Chapter 7 apply here as well – good diet, exercise, healthy weight, etc.

Avoid or limit infections. Practice good personal hygiene. Avoid dry skin by applying lotions. Even an infection from an insect bite can lead to lymphedema. Don't be cavalier about small wounds – clean them carefully, keep covered, and use a topical antibiotic until wound is healed. If after a couple of days the wound gets worse, reddens, is painful or is accompanied by a fever, contact a health care professional. Infection avoidance is especially important in the elderly or those with weak immune systems.

Symptoms

- Swelling of a limb or body part, usually arm, hand, legs, and/or feet

- Sensations of heaviness, tightness or numbness

- Skin feeling tight

- Decreased flexibility in the hand, wrist or ankle

Course if untreated

The lymph vessels can deteriorate until flow is perhaps just 20% of a healthy system before any symptoms appear. Damage is occurring without any outward sign, except some patients feel "heaviness".

Eventually, however, the damage is so great that the lymph vessels begin to expand from the increased volume of fluids with nowhere to go. The valves separate, allowing pooling at the bottom of the affected limb or tissue (usually the feet and hands). The limb becomes heavy. In the beginning the condition is mostly painless. If only one limb is affected, it's clearly larger than the other.

An inflammatory process begins, destroying the elastic fibers and filling the extracellular space with collagen. This begins the non-pitting edema stage. Local immune functions are disturbed resulting in infections.

The skin thickens. At first it looks like the skin of an orange but then it hardens further, often darkening. The skin is prone to splitting, inviting infection. Also, the split skin can release lymph, which irritates the skin.

Lymphedema is divided into at least four stages:

Stage	Appearance/Symptoms

0	• A limb may feel heavy at times but there is no measureable swelling • Bioimpedence and other diagnostic tests can be used to establish baselines for high-risk surgical patients as well as to monitor suspected impending lymphedema. • This can be a reversible stage if diagnosed
1	• Edema is pitting – pushing a finger into it will leave an impression. Edema often starts with end of limb – foot or hand. Edema is reversible, relieved by elevation. • This can be reversed
2	• Edema in non-pitting, fibrosis has begun. This means there is hardening within extracellular spaces. • Treatable but not reversible
3	• Called the "lymphostatic elephantiasis" stage. Limb or tissue has become irreversibly hardened. Limbs become huge. • Some have proposed a Stage 4 in which the limb has no pulse even with ultrasound and the skin is so brittle it breaks if tapped.

Complications of Lymphedema include:

- A major complication of chronic lymphedema is lymph cancers. After 10 years of lymphedema, patients have a 10% risk of lymphangiosarcoma, which is an aggressive cancer requiring amputation if possible, and often fatal. Other cancers also occur as a complication.
- Bacterial and fungal infections. These can become systemic. Gangrene can occur.
- Pain. Pain pressure on nerves as well as from infections or irritation from lymph on the skin.
- Loss of function of the affected limb or tissue
- Depression
- Joint pain from the weight
- Lungs. If the lymph system in the chest and abdomen are affected, fluid builds up in the lungs.
- Amputation.

Diagnosis

When lymphedema is already present, the diagnosis is usually made from taking a history and performing a physical exam. However, tests are often needed to detect its specific cause, the degree of lymph damage, and to measure the degree of swelling that's already occurred.

If lymphedema can be predicted, patient education is important. For patients undergoing breast surgery for example, educating them about the potential of lymphedema has been show to lead to earlier diagnosis and treatment resulting in improved outcomes.

Stage the degree of swelling to act as baseline: for patients undergoing breast surgery, simple measurements of the arm(s) prior to surgery and then making follow-up measurements can help detect patients early in the disease process.

Treatments

For all patients, the earlier the diagnosis, the better the outcome – IF a lifetime of careful and often tedious routines are followed. One of the first steps is to find health care professionals that have been trained in the care of lymphedema.

It's important that patients do not self-diagnose and try to self-treat with compression tapes or garments. In addition, physicians untrained in lymph diseases may casually prescribe the wrong treatment. The wrong type or strength of compression products can cause irreparable damage to the lymph system – or not be effective at all, allowing progression of the disease. Similarly, massage or other treatments even by professionals who have not been trained in lymph treatments should be avoided.

Treatment approaches include meticulous skin hygiene, avoiding trauma, wearing pressure garments or bandages, physical therapy, directed exercise. Some pharmaceuticals and skin creams are beneficial. Surgery techniques abound and some have now been shown to be effective.

Skin care

The National Cancer Institute's PDQ summary for lymphedema provides a detailed and helpful list of precautions to take in caring for the skin of an affected limb:

- Use cream or lotion to keep the skin moist.
- Treat small cuts or breaks in the skin with an antibacterial ointment.
- Avoid needle sticks of any type into the limb (arm or leg) with lymphedema. This includes shots or blood tests.
- Use a thimble for sewing.
- Avoid testing bath or cooking water using the limb with lymphedema. There may be less feeling (touch, temperature, pain) in the affected arm or leg, and skin might burn in water that is too hot.
- Wear gloves when gardening and cooking.
- Wear sunscreen and shoes when outdoors.
- Cut toenails straight across. See a podiatrist as needed to prevent ingrown nails and infections.
- Keep feet clean and dry and wear cotton socks.

Physical therapy

The goal of physical therapy is to stimulate lymph drainage without causing damage. Various techniques are used to coax the excess fluid out of the tissues, including gentle hand massage or mechanical pumps. Then special bandages or compression garments are worn to keep fluid from rebounding. Usually many treatments are given initially by a therapist until most of the fluid has been removed, then patients are taught to do most of the care themselves at home.

Treatment is given by therapists trained in this specialty. The massages are gentle and follow lymph anatomy. When the swelling is still liquid or not yet apparent (Stage 0 and 1) the swelling is reduced over a period of a few weeks with massage and wrappings. When the swelling has been stabilized, measurements for compression garments are made and these are worn either overnight or all day at home.

At home, sometimes caution and exercise is sufficient. Other patients must do daily self-massage, wear constrictive garments, and/or use mechanical pumps. Care can take 1-2 hours a day.

Mechanical pumps

Mechanical pumps are prescribed by physicians. They involve fitting garments that deliver directional air pressure to the body. Garments may be fitted over an arm or leg or include the trunk as well. If the pressure is not fixed by the manufacturer, patients are warned not to increase the pressure beyond that being prescribed. As with human massage, heavy pressure is not better pressure and can harm the lymphatics and surrounding already damaged tissue. Most insurance companies provide reimbursement for the pumps, although they often delay approval by requiring patients try other solutions.

Compression garments

Compression on the outside of a limb supports the muscles and increases lymph flow. The amount and direction of compression are important and are prescribed by physicians and fitted by lymphedema therapist for all but the mildest cases. Compression products have a wide range of fabrics and padding and are made in many forms that are easy (or at least easier) for the patient to put on. Pressures range from 20-60 mmHg.

Compression garments or bandages can be over-the-counter generic products in a few sizes or custom made. Often premade garments are recommended for those at risk of lymphedema, such as those undergoing breast surgery. These would be available if any swelling of the arm is detected. Later, other garments may be recommended if the edema is not reversed early. Some insurances pay for a limited number of specially formed garments but will not pay for the others. Some US states have laws now that require insurance coverage. Medicare does not yet formally reimburse for any compression garments, but some patients have received it; The Lymphedema Treatment Act introduced in several sessions would provide this coverage but has not been passed.

Garments can be expensive, especially if needed to be worn day and night. Night garments can run at $300-2000/£200-1600. Daytime garments can run from $50-300/£33-200 or more and require replacing 2-4 times a year. These estimates are for a single arm or leg; chest/trunk or multiple limb involvement will increase the cost considerably.

Exercise

The best results for patients with lymphedema are from maintaining a healthy body weight and being as fit as possible.

Those at risk of and/or who actually have lymphedema have been shown to benefit from walking, jogging, and swimming. Years ago patients thought to be at risk for lymphedema were warned to avoid exercise but studies have shown it to be safe. Patients recovering from surgery or radiation that puts them at risk also benefit from range of motion exercises to maintain tendon health and to avoid adhesions.

Those with lymphedema benefit from specific exercises as part of an overall treatment program. These are sometimes called lymph remedial exercises and are similar to tai chi in that they include slow, low impact, and repetitive motions. Unlike tai chi, they are performed with compression garments or wraps (or performed in a swimming pool), and movements are designed specifically to improve lymph circulation in the affected areas. The exercises increase repetitions and activity slowly and if a higher level is not maintained for a week or so, the patient has to start again at a lower level to avoid damage.

A person should be guided in the choice of exercise by someone trained in lymphedema therapy. The website for the Lymphology Association of North America maintains a worldwide list of certified therapists.

Pharmaceuticals and Natural Supplements

Drug therapy is not a major component of treatment. Aside from the anthelminthics or antibacterial/antifungal medications, most treatment guidelines for the disease do not recommend many medicines as proven effective and urge caution if trying a natural supplement.

Anthelminthics: Diagnosis of nematode-caused lymphedema can now be made by testing a drop of blood for antibodies to the worm. Several drugs can treat the disease and prevent the lymphatic damage if diagnosed early enough. The World Health Organization and others are now attempting to eradicate the worm by treating entire populations with drugs for several years and drug companies are donating the medicines. This erases the worm from the area's mosquitos. Treating much of the population once a year with two medications has been found effective. Drug combinations have been albendazole plus either diethylcarbamazine citrate (DEC) or ivermectin. In some areas these drugs have been added to common household table salt used by the community.

Antibacterials/antifungals: Patients are prone to bacterial or fungal infections, especially those with more damaged skin. Diagnosed early, often topical medication is effective; oral drugs are given as needed. Patients who have experienced repeated bouts of cellulitis or other persistent infections are placed on long-term or preventive medication.

Diuretics: Diuretics are not useful for removing the protein-laden interstitial fluid of lymphedema. While they may attract some water from the fluid, the proteins will just draw it back in. Diuretics may cause dehydration, electrolyte problems, or damage tissues.

If diuretics must be used for other medical conditions, the patient's blood chemistry is carefully monitored to be sure electrolytes such as potassium, magnesium, and sodium are in proper balance. This is no trivial concern: much of the body's function depends upon different levels of each electrolyte being on opposite sides of a cell wall – these differences regulate fluid balance, acidity, nerve conduction, muscle contraction, and blood pressure – just to list a few.

Retinoids: Retinoids are applied directly to the affected skin or taken orally, and are effective in advancing lymphedema to soften the affected skin or prevent keratinization. The skin is then less vulnerable to infection and inflammatory processes. These drugs are related to Vitamin A, were developed to treat psoriasis, and can't be taken by pregnant women as they cause birth defects. An oral drug is acitretin. Tazorotene is a topical medication.

Benzopyrones/flavonoids: These antioxidant plant substances include coumarin and grape seed oil. They are thought to bind with proteins and help cause their breakdown. Coumarin especially has been used in the past for lymphedema in tandem with physical therapies; some find it effective if taken for a long time as it acts very slowly. So far most clinical trials have not proved its effectiveness. In addition, coumarin is toxic to the liver in 5-10% of patients – thought to be the result of genetic differences. If it doesn't reduce the swelling from lymphedema, it is said by many to stabilize it. Coumarin has been banned by the US Food and Drug Administration as a food additive since 1950. (Coumarin is often confused with the blood thinner Coumadin (a brand name for warfarin) – even in medical literature.)

Proteases: Proteases are compounds that break up proteins. Some are harvested from animal pancreas and bile; other sources are from fruits such as pineapple and papaya. These have been used for lymphedema and are being activity studied. Their action is comparable to benzopyrones in that they are break up fibrin and other proteins in an affected area. Proteases being studied are those taken orally and applied to the affected areas.

Oral sodium selenite was shown to have some effect for arm and head/neck lymphedema.

Oral extracts of the American horse chestnut seed have been effective for treating venous insufficiency (failed valves and leaking walls); while suggested for treating lymphedema it has not been effective.

Lymph growth factors: This is a promising area of research. Various growth factors are being studied, including stem cells, to encourage the regrowth of damaged lymphatics. So far, studies show the growth of components but not restoration of a functioning lymphatic system.

Surgery

Surgical procedures used today are mainly those to debulk diseased tissue – to reduce the size of the limb so it is more functional and less vulnerable to infections. Sequential or single step approaches are taken and involve removing the skin and all or much of the subcutaneous tissue from the limb. The limb is either immediately or within a week or so grafted with a portion of the removed skin.

Most of the other surgical procedures are still in a research stage. One that is used clinically now is connecting the lymph system to a healthy venous system, if one exists in the limb. This lymph/venous connective microsurgery is also done during extensive pelvic surgery for cancer. Success has been found to be dependent upon patient selection (early in the disease) and meticulous surgical and postsurgical care. Other surgical procedures being used include transplanting lymph nodes and vessels and liposuction.

Low Power (Cold) Laser

Lasers are used in conjunction with other therapies, not by themselves. Studies have shown results varying from 1-30% reduction in volume of a limb. Arms respond better to lasers than legs. Lasers' place in treatment of lymphedema is still under review. Most insurance companies consider lasers experimental and do not reimburse for their use.

The US Food and Drug Administration has approved the use of low level lasers for treating lymphedema. These lasers deliver red or near-infrared light. The lights delivered are poorly absorbed so penetrate deeply. The more commonly used laser in clinical studies delivers a 904 nm light that is not visible and produces no heat. The light is thought to stimulate lymph flow and the growth of new lymph vessels as well as break up scar tissue and prevent scar tissue from adhering to healthy tissue. The action of the laser is believed to be through stimulation of mitochondria within cells. (Mitochondria are sort of like batteries.)

The laser has been studied mostly in post mastectomy patients and has shown positive results in some clinical trials, with small but significant improvement. Handheld, battery powered lasers are available for purchase by patients; these should be used with guidance of therapist and physician. The 904 nm lasers are expensive ($4000/£2600 plus); lower nm lasers to 600 nm are a fraction of the cost and may be effective. Some companies rent the equipment and sell used machines.

Hyperbaric oxygen was studied in the UK and found to have little or no value.

Groups
There are several websites that provide reams of practical information and also respond to individual questions. Most are also involved in lobbying. Among them are:

- Lymphedema People.
  www.**lymphedemapeople**.com
  Good information overall – especially of insurance issues
- Step Up, Speak Out.
  www.**stepup-speakout**.org
  Good review of new therapies – what to watch out for. Also excellent paper on things you want your doctor to be. Another paper "Essential Lymphedema Information for All Health Care

Providers: from a Physician with Secondary Lymphedema"
was written by a physician dismayed by the lack of physician
training and knowledge of lymphedema.

- Lymphology Association of North America.
  www.clt-**lana**.org
  Has worldwide list of certified lymphedema therapists
- National Lymphedema Network.
  www.lymphnet.org
  Has some information on website. Membership (paid) needed
  for newsletters and some publications.
- Lymphoedema Support Network.
  www.**lymphoedema**.org
  UK organization of healthcare professional and patients.
  Memberships are free; the organization charges clinics for
  some printed materials.

Barriers to care

Successful care of lymphedema depends on a correct and early
diagnosis, prompt and correct treatment, and patient adherence to
the treatment plan. Patients report obstacles to all of these.
Patients are often told the swelling will go away by itself.
Inappropriate treatments have included diuretics and regular
punishing physical therapy. Barriers to a patient's adherence to a
correct treatment plan include access to therapist, cost of care and
supplies, discomfort of the treatment, and the effort and/or time
needed to stick to a plan. Education prior to cancer surgery to
spark early diagnosis has been found effective in studies but not
often given. Education about the disease and the dangers of its
progression is often lacking once the disease is diagnosed. One
woman stated her reason for sticking to her compression garments
and exercises was seeing someone with advanced disease at the
clinic.

CHAPTER 8: WATER RETENTION IN A SINGLE ORGAN: THE BRAIN

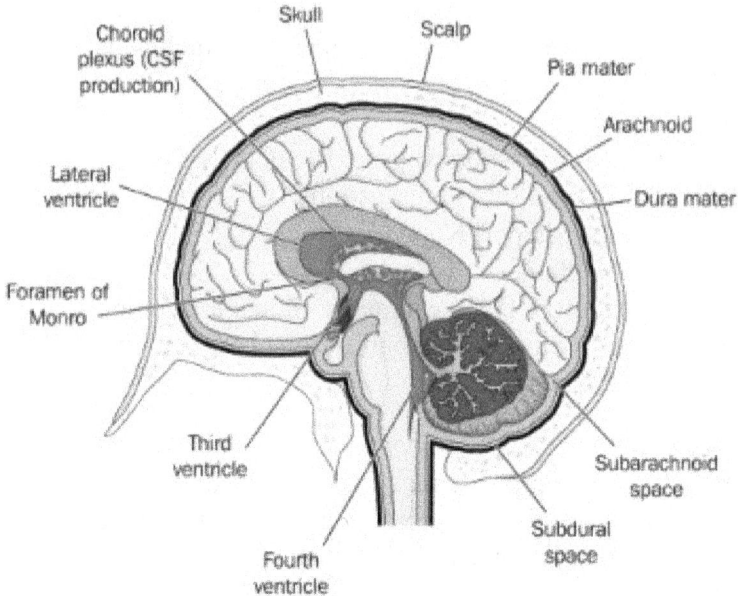

Picture: The Brain

The brain is enclosed on most sides by bone. To protect the brain from crashing into the skull bone when we move, it's cushioned by cerebrospinal fluid both around the outside in the subarachnoid and subdural spaces and within its ventricles. Usually the brain is protected from excess fluids by the blood brain barrier, as substances such as salt and proteins cannot pass easily into the brain and draw water in with them. Any excess fluid in the brain can disrupt this cocooning and increase pressure on brain cells, causing temporary or permanent damage. This swelling is called cerebral edema.

Blood does not circulate into the brain as it does in most organs. The endothelium of capillaries near the brain are joined tightly together to form tubes that don't allow most molecules into the brain. The way substances pass through the barrier are either directly through the endothelial membrane or by active transport. The membrane is made of fat so that small fat-soluble substances such as some barbiturates can pass through. Water, some gases (oxygen, carbon dioxide, and anesthesia gases), alcohol, nicotine, and some viruses can also pass through. Other molecules are carried through the membrane by specific transport proteins in the endothelium; for example, these have been developed to transport glucose into the brain for energy and sodium and chlorine ions. The barrier protects the brain but also makes treatment of any infections difficult, as most drugs won't pass through the barrier.

The blood brain barrier was discovered 100 years ago by Ehrlich and Goldman when they injected water-soluble blue dyes into a vein of an animal and found that while most of its organs turned blue, the brain (except for a few small areas at its base) and the spinal cord and spinal fluid did not. Later it was discovered that as the endothelium is made of largely fat, small fat-soluble substances like alcohol could pass through easily. Much later the active transport systems were discovered.

What can cause the blood brain barrier to fail?

The tight connections between endothelial cells can be disrupted.

This can be caused by trauma to the head, brain tumors, high blood pressure, infections, and restriction of blood supply to the brain. There is also a severe form of altitude sickness that can occur after a week or so at unaccustomed high altitude. It is believed that this long period of low oxygen affects the endothelial cells and they begin to leak.

The active transport proteins are damaged

The endothelial cells remain tightly joined but the sodium and potassium active transport pump is damaged, allowing excess ions into the brain bringing water with them. This can be caused by poisons, serious cardiac events, and ischemic strokes (strokes caused by blockage of a brain vessel). Reye's syndrome can also cause this; Reye's is a mysterious, sudden illness that occurs during recovery of a viral illness when taking aspirin or other oral or topical salicylate.

Circulating plasma is diluted

Usually there is more "stuff" in plasma than in the cerebrospinal fluid or the extracellular fluid of the brain. This keeps excess water from being attracted into the brain. When plasma becomes more dilute than brain fluids, the situation reverses and water is attracted into the brain.

Excess water alone can cause this. Excessive intake is one way this happens. Or excess water can be retained in the body by abnormally high levels of antidiuretic hormone (ADH). ADH stops the kidney from releasing water. Many things can increase ADH including a wide variety of cancers, multiple sclerosis, infections such as tuberculosis, trauma, surgery, and Guillian-Barré Syndrome

The drug ecstasy can cause cerebral edema from two directions: it increases ADH and often the people who take this drug feel thirsty and drink huge amounts of water.

Low levels of substances in plasma can also be a trigger, pulling water from plasma into the brain. A sudden drop in glucose for example, as in a complication of treating diabetes, or from alcohol, starvation, infections, and organ failure can cause brain swelling. Low levels of sodium in plasma (hyponatremia) can also lead to brain swelling. This is caused by extreme endurance sports, surgical fluid imbalance, and as a complication of liver or heart failure.

Cerebrospinal fluid circulation is blocked

About 20-25 oz. (600-700 ml) of cerebral spinal fluid (CSF) is produced within the adult brain every day. Most of it flows out into the venous or lymphatic system. Only 5-9 oz. (140-270 ml) remains in the brain and spinal column at any one time. If there is blockage either within the brain cavities or surrounding it, pressure will build. If not relieved, the CSF will infiltrate the interstitial space, causing edema.

Causes of the blockage include developmental disorder, infection, tumor, or cerebral aneurysm.

Another result of CSF being blocked is hydrocephalus, a condition in which the ventricles enlarge. Hydrocephalus is discussed separately in the chapter on third spaces.

What are the symptoms of cerebral edema?

Symptoms may develop suddenly or slowly depending upon the cause and the area of the brain first affected. Headache, neck pain, nausea, vomiting, dizziness, confusion, and vision changes are among the more common early symptoms. Pupils may not be equal or react differently to light. Loss of consciousness, seizures, or coma may follow if the edema is not reversed. Respiratory problems or respiratory arrest may occur if the swelling squeezes the lower brain stem.

How is cerebral edema diagnosed?

Much of the diagnosis depends upon the physician having a good history of what's happened with the patient, including the speed of any changes that have occurred. This is followed by a physical exam, including a neurological exam, to determine if the brain is truly affected and what parts of it may be involved.
Level of consciousness, speech, cranial nerves, strength, balance and deep tendon reflexes are all evaluated.

Finding the cause of the edema is not simple. The blood pressure is monitored and blood tests may provide clues if low sodium or glucose is suspected. MRI and CT exams can give anatomical details of what may be happening. Pressure within a brain ventricle is monitored in special units of acute care hospitals. Spinal fluid pressure is sometimes used to estimate intracranial pressure but is usually avoided as release of fluid from the spine creates a pressure gradient and may draw the lower brain structures against the skull and damage them.

Treatment of cerebral edema

Much of the treatment depends upon treating the root cause of the problem. Slight cases of edema may resolve on their own without treatment but with careful observation. More serious cases need to be handled quickly to avoid long-term brain damage or death.

Treatments are aimed at reducing the edema and keeping well-oxygenated blood circulating to the brain. If hypernatremia is the root cause, mannitol or a highly concentrated IV sodium chloride solution is given to attract excess water from the brain.

If the brain swelling and high cerebral fluid pressure cannot be reversed quickly enough, sometimes a surgical approach is taken; either tapping any excess fluid from the brain ventricles or by removing part of the skull to allow the brain to expand without increasing pressure.

Can cerebral edema be prevented?
Trauma is a major cause of cerebral edema. To prevent this, wear helmets for sports, biking and motorcycling and wear seat belts when in a vehicle.

Avoid high blood pressure and heart disease if you can and make lifestyle changes and take medications if you have them.

Be alert if anyone has symptoms of cerebral edema when at high altitudes. We can drive to areas that can trigger both cerebral and pulmonary (lung) edema. Mountain safety experts recommend that once climbers are above 10,000 feet (3000 meters) that each night they not increase their altitude for sleeping by more than 1500 feet over the previous night. Now in the US you can drive right up to the top of Mt. Evans in Colorado, which is at 14,240 feet.

The most important message of this chapter is to listen to the experts. If anyone has been hit in the head, follow instructions. If you live alone and were told to wake up every hour or two to check for symptoms, get someone to help. Don't shrug it off. If you have a disease that can lead to brain damage from edema, follow the treatments you've been prescribed. All too often people die or are permanently brain damaged by having a cavalier attitude towards treatment.

CHAPTER 9: WATER RETENTION IN A SINGLE ORGAN: PULMONARY EDEMA

Breathing adds oxygen (O_2) to the blood and removes carbon dioxide (CO_2). This exchange of gases is done in the lung between capillaries and alveoli, both having very thin walls. The body's 300,000 alveoli, also known as air sacks, are the end points of the bronchial tubes and are surrounded by capillaries. Most of the alveoli are arranged in bunches – much like grapes.

Between the capillaries and alveoli is the interstitial space, which is sometimes very thin and contains a fluid low in protein (so it doesn't suck fluid from the capillaries). The gases flow through the interstitial space to make exchanges. The direction of gas flow is from highest concentration to lowest, so CO_2 flows out of the capillaries coming from the body as O_2 flows into them from the alveoli. In a normal lung, very little fluid escapes the capillaries as they are more tightly connected than elsewhere in the body.

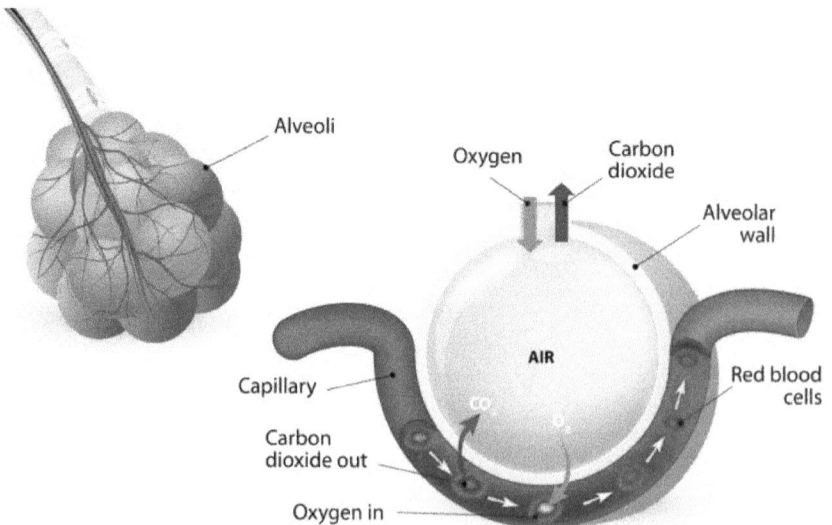

Picture: Alveoli in a clump and the exchange of gasses with lung capillaries

In pulmonary edema, excess fluid may be in the air sacs or in the surrounding lung tissue itself. The edema is usually from an increase in the pressure of blood within the lungs, causing the capillaries to leak. The fluid reduces the ability of the lungs to exchange oxygen and carbon dioxide from the blood vessels to the air. Pulmonary edema can lead to respiratory failure.

Symptoms of pulmonary edema may include:

- Difficulty breathing. At night it may be difficult for patients to lie flat in bed or they may have scary episodes of breathlessness.
- Coughing up blood, often pink foam
- A feeling of suffocating or drowning
- Wheezing or gasping for breath
- Anxiety
- Chest pain
- An irregularly fast heartbeat
- Problems speaking in full sentences because of shortness of breath
- Excessive sweating
- If the lung edema is caused by a failing left ventricle of the heart, the legs and liver may also be swollen.

What causes pulmonary edema?

The causes are usually explained as either heart-related or having other, non-heart causes.

When the heart is the culprit

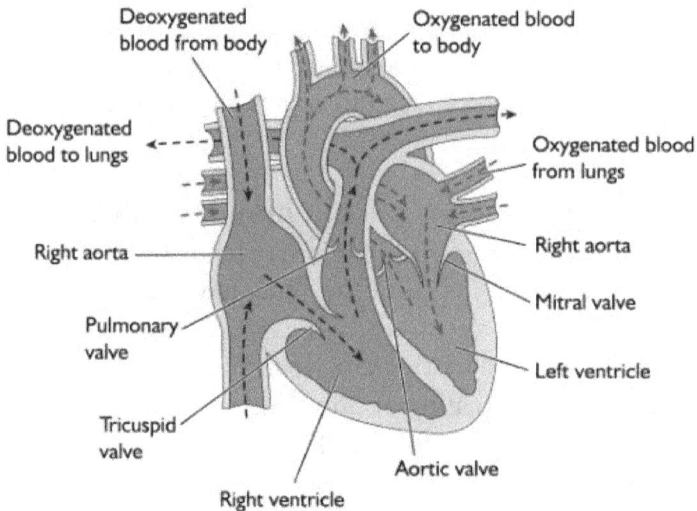

Picture: Blood flow through the heart

First, a quick trip around the body's blood circulation:

- Blood high in CO_2 returns from the body, flows into the right atrium then the right ventricle where it is pumped into the lungs where it becomes oxygenated.
- Blood rich in O_2 flows from the lungs into the left atrium then the left ventricle and pumped out to the body.
- The walls of the right ventricle are thin and the blood pressure to the lungs fairly low – systolic pressure ranges from 15 to 30 mmHg. When oxygenated blood reaches the left ventricle the pressure is very low, from 2 to 15 mmHg. The walls of the left ventricle are thick and deliver the blood through the arteries at fairly high pressures – with systolic pressure ranging from 120 to 140 mmHg.

So why does the heart cause lung edema?

Under normal circumstances, the capillaries in the lung are tightly joined and very little fluid escapes into the lung's interstitial spaces. This is aided by the low pressure of blood in the lungs and the low osmotic pressure of the surrounding intracellular spaces. When the heart fails, blood backs up in the lungs, increasing the blood pressure there. Sovari (2014) describes the three stages of what happens next in the lungs when lung pressure and pressure in the left atrium increases.

Stage 1. The increased blood pressure in the lungs at first widens already-opened lung blood vessels and then opens the smaller ones. The exchange of gases may actually improve at this stage.

Stage 2. Fluid now leaks from the distended capillaries into the interstitial space. At first, the lymphatics take up the extra fluid. When the lymphatics are overwhelmed, the increased pressure in the interstitial space may collapse some of the small airways called bronchioles. (The trachea splits into two bronchial tubes, which then branch off to smaller and smaller airways. The large bronchi have cartilage rings or plates to keep them open. When the "tree" gets to the level of the air sacs the bronchioles depend upon connection to surrounding tissue to keep them open). Symptoms of low blood oxygen (hypoxemia) may be evident at this stage.

Stage 3. The interstitial spaces are all filled with fluid so the fluid starts to leak into the alveoli. This leads to severe hypoxemia and symptoms are noticeable. An inflammatory process is often involved which disrupts the membranes of both capillaries and alveoli.

What's wrong with the heart that causes this?

A number of things can go wrong with the heart that lead to pulmonary edema, including:

Obstruction of the left atrium. This backs up blood coming from the lungs and is often caused by the narrowing of the mitral valve from rheumatic fever or by failure of a replacement valve.

Defect of left ventricle. This is the body's pump, when it starts to fail the body reacts by increasing fluid volume, which increases fluid pressure. Heart attacks, patients going off low salt diets or not taking prescribed diuretics, anemia, chronic valve disorders, and toxins (alcohol, some illegal drugs, and some medicines) can all affect the ventricle.

Fluid overload. Some kidney problems and excess IV fluid administrations can increase overall fluid pressure.

Rupture of part of the heart from trauma or heart attack.

Other. Sudden increases in very high blood pressure, new attacks of rapid heartbeat, obstructions anywhere in the heart, and heart failure can result in pulmonary edema.

What are the non-heart related causes?

Non-cardiac causes of pulmonary edema range from direct injury to the lung to a complication of a systemic infection and include:

Upper airway obstruction. Pulmonary edema can occur after an obstruction is relieved, either by removing an object or from surgery such as that for swollen tonsils and adenoids. In young, strong men it is thought to be caused by their extreme efforts to breathe, which creates a negative pressure, increasing venous return to the lung while decreasing cardiac output. The pulmonary edema after surgery is confusing and may have multiple causes.

Nervous system causes. Pulmonary edema may occur after a seizure, severe electric shock, strangulation, or head injury. Lung edema may result from nervous system disorder causing increased tone of the atrium and/or constriction of the lung vessels; other pathways are also possible.

Injury to the lungs. Injuries can disrupt the whole structure of the lung or attack the membranes between capillaries and air sacks. Injuries can include strong physical forces, such as those in an automobile accident or inhaling hot air or toxins such as chlorine or ammonia.

Infections. Viral infections such as Hantavirus and dengue fever cause fatal lung edemas.

Inhaling vomit.

Blood clots. Blood clots from deep veins travel to the lungs and lodge in a lung vessel. Damage from the loss of circulation to part of the lung can result in edema. Large clots in the lung cause the more familiar pulmonary embolism, an acute condition that can be fatal.

Smoke from a fire. Breathing heavy smoke can damage the membranes of capillaries and air sacks leading to lung edema.

Drugs and Medicines. Rarely, heroin and cocaine can cause lung edema. Aspirin poisoning can do this as well; this occurs among the elderly who take aspirin continually.

Swimming. Swimming-induced pulmonary edema happens in vigorous water sports. How it happens isn't clear yet. Near drowning can also cause lung edema.

High altitude pulmonary edema. This can happen at altitudes over 8,000 feed (2400 m). It usually occurs after a few days for those unaccustomed to high altitudes, but it can also happen to those who've been up high for a while but who exercise more than usual. This also causes cerebral edema.

What is acute respiratory distress syndrome or ARDS?

ARDS is a subset of non-cardiac pulmonary edema. It often occurs among patients who are already in hospital. ARDS is characterized by sudden failure of the respiratory system for which clinicians have trouble providing adequate oxygen. It can occur 1-3 days after an injury (which includes some surgeries) or infection. Inflammation disturbs the membranes of both capillaries and alveoli allowing flooding of the air sacks.

There are perhaps 200,000 ARDS patients a year in the US. Mortality can be high, 25%-40%, but used to be much higher. Death is often from multiple organ failure from lack of oxygen. One treatment which has reduced mortality is adjusting ventilators to deliver smaller breaths than usually given to pulmonary patients.

Diagnosis

The patient with acute pulmonary edema is in distress and usually seen in the emergency room or hospital. When the diagnosis has been made and the cause known, some patients are considered to have the risk of chronic pulmonary edema and followed by primary care physicians or by specialists to avoid future acute episodes.

The diagnosis is made by taking a full history and physical exam and evaluating the results of some tests.

A plain chest x-ray provides a clue of whether the edema is heart-related or not. Further radiologic tests such as ultrasound, CT and MRI may follow. The acute patients may have both cardiac and non-cardiac edemas at the same time.

Blood O_2 and CO_2 are determined first using noninvasive sensors. Arterial blood may be taken as it gives additional information. Other blood tests are ordered depending upon the diagnoses being considered.

A culture of sputum and other fluids if infections are suspected.

Bronchoscopy. This is direct viewing of the lungs.

ECG. An electrocardiogram may also provide additional information about the heart.

Treatment

Oxygen is given right away – either through a facemask, nasal cannula, or for infants, enclosures of several types. If needed, oxygen may be delivered by a ventilator through an opening made in the trachea.

Diuretics to remove excess fluids from the body, including the lung, may be given after the cause of the edema has been established.

Various drugs to counter underlying heart conditions are given when the diagnosis is established. As noted elsewhere, many of the patients will have known heart conditions except for those with a first heart attack.

Prevention

Many acute cases of cardiac-related pulmonary edema result from the worsening of known heart disease or from poor compliance with medications and dietary changes or exercise prescribed for it. The prevention of heart disease follows the same guidelines outlined in the chapter on vascular health.

Non-cardiac pulmonary edema has so many initial causes that prevention is pretty much a warning to stay as healthy as you can. Younger patients do better than older ones, which isn't controllable. Obesity may be a factor. Alcohol abuse is a factor in both incidence and survival of ARDS. The use of cocaine and heroin, and chronic use of aspirin can be avoided.

Note: Pleural effusion is fluid that is under the outside lining of the lungs and described in the chapter on third spacing.

CHAPTER 10: EXTREME "THIRD SPACING"

Third spacing sounds like something out of science fiction, but it's a medical term concerning the movement of fluids in the body. The term "third space" is used to distinguish spaces where fluid doesn't normally collect in large amounts. In addition, third space fluid doesn't communicate easily with blood vessels to return its fluid into general circulation – so once it's in the third space there are difficulties getting it out.

Before going further, let's refresh the basics from Chapter 1: most (about 67%) of the water in the body is intracellular – fluid inside individual cells. Plasma and lymph account for another 5%, interstitial fluid is around 15%, and the various compartments, 2-3%. Interstitial fluid is the fluid found *between* cells *inside* an organ – like the lungs, brain, and skin. The compartments may be those that surround an organ like the lungs or be large spaces like the peritoneal cavity, the space filled with the abdominal organs.

Single organ third spacing includes cerebral edema and pulmonary edema. Angioedema and anaphylaxis are examples of third spacing with fluid escaping into interstitial spaces. Compartmental third space disorders include hydrocephalus, pleural effusion, ascites, and anasarca. Cerebral and pulmonary edema are discussed in separate chapters. The third spacing conditions discussed in this chapter are: angioedema, anaphylaxis, hydrocephalus, pleural effusion, ascites, and anasarca.

A. Angioedema

We are all familiar with hives; the round, raised, itching welts that can occur on the skin. The medical term for hives is urticaria. The fluid in the welts comes from leaking capillaries and common causes of hives are allergies, tension, and insect bites.

Angioedema is a similar condition but occurs within the deeper layers of the skin, the fat under the skin, mucous membranes, and tissues under the mucous membranes (The mucous membranes are linings similar to skin but are inside the body including mouth, nose, and urinary and digestive tracts).

The chemicals that cause the capillaries to leak are histamines in allergy-related cases and bradykinins in many of the others. Angioedema can affect any part of the body, but usually affects the eyes, face, mouth and throat, hands, feet, and genitals. Perhaps 10-20% of the population has experienced at least one episode of this, with 0.5% having recurring attacks. Almost half of people also have welts on the skin's surface at the same time.

There are basically two forms of angioedema, a type caused by a genetic dysfunction and the other type. The most critical medical emergency that occurs in both types is the blocking of the airway from swollen tissues in the mouth and throat.

Non-hereditary angioedema

This edema occurs rapidly and most often in the face. If the skin is affected, the patients may feel heat and pain but no itching unless they have hives. The skin may be slightly pink. If the eyes are involved, vision may be obscured. The swellings may last up to three days.

Triggers

Allergies. Common allergies are to foods, dyes, pollens, insect bites, and latex. Sometimes aspirin (or other NSAIDs like Aleve) and penicillin can cause angioedema. Often allergies to NSAIDs are accompanied with allergies to the food coloring such as yellow dye no. 5.

Foods that can trigger an attack include nuts, dairy products (mostly from cow's milk), seafood, legumes and their oils (peanuts, tree nuts, soy, beans, peas, lentils, flour containing lupine), citrus fruit, eggs, wheat, chocolate, licorice, berries, and cinnamon.

Medicines. Medicine-caused angioedema is rare, but the drugs most often implicated are the ACE inhibitors prescribed for high blood pressure. The drug reaction may not occur until the patient has been taking it for several years so it is difficult to diagnose. Angioedema episodes may also persist long after the medicine is stopped. Common ACE inhibitors include benazepril (Lotensin); captopril (Capoten); and enalapril maleate (Vasotec). Angiotensin II type I receptor blockers (ARBs) used to treat heart failure have also been shown to cause angioedemas. These drugs include candesartan (Atacand); eprosartan (Teveten; irbesartan (Avapro); and losartan (Cozaar)

Suspected causes. Angioedema may be a result of infections, stress or anxiety, tight clothes, strenuous exercise, alcohol, or heat. Thyroid conditions and vitamin deficiencies have also been suspected.

Treatment

Airway obstruction is a medical emergency and the most serious risk in angioedema. Passing a tube to the lungs through the mouth or a surgical opening in the neck may be needed to provide oxygen while waiting for medicines to work. If angioedema had an allergic cause, treatment with epinephrine is used to restore the airway. Anti-inflammatory medicines (corticosteroids) and antihistamines are also given; if the airway is not involved, these may be the only medicines needed.

If the angioedema is not caused by an allergic reaction, the treatments used for allergy patients are not terribly effective. This is especially true of the ACE and ABS related conditions. Higher doses of corticosteroids with the antihistamine drugs may reduce the need for (or the length of) intubation, and the length of hospital stays. Fresh frozen plasma has had some success.

Prevention

Prevention first involves the avoidance of the triggering substances or situations. If the allergen is known, a series of desensitizing injections with increasing amounts of it may be needed if the angioedema symptoms are severe. If the cause of the condition is the ACE or ABS medication, other treatments for high blood pressure are substituted. Patients at risk of airway obstruction are given epinephrine (such as the Epipen) to administer themselves and told to then seek urgent medical care after using it. Other patients are told how to use antihistamines. Identifying bracelets are also lifesaving as they can alert caregivers if the patient isn't able to communicate.

Hot water makes swelling worse, so should be avoided. Cold water may relieve symptoms; many patients learn to enjoy the relief that cold showers or baths give them.

Complications

Death by asphyxiation is the more common, serious complication of angioedema. In addition, patients with allergic angioedema also have a risk of anaphylaxis, a severe and potentially fatal condition also described in this chapter.

Hereditary angioedema

Hereditary angioedema (HAE) is a rare, serious form of recurrent angioedema and affects an estimated one in 10,000 to 50,000 people worldwide. The condition is autosomal dominant: if one parent carries the gene, each birth will have a 50% chance of having the disease. It is thought that perhaps 20% of cases occur spontaneously without known inheritance and that it happens at conception. The genetic disorder has over 200 mutations.

Patients may have their first episode from one year old to their early forties, with about 75% coming before age fifteen.

Symptoms generally begin with mild swellings that become more severe around the time of puberty. Sex and race don't seem to be overwhelming factors in the occurrence of HAE, except women may have more serious attacks. Many of the patients also have an autoimmune disease in addition to HAE.

Swelling can be dramatic; swollen faces can be unrecognizable. Almost all HAE patients experience episodes of skin and intestinal swelling. Besides being disfiguring, swelling of the hands, feet, mouth, and eyes often prevent patients from normal activities. Patients often are disabled for 100 or more days each year. There are no hives associated with HAE but about a third of patients feel tingling or have a red rash before the onset.

Swelling of the intestinal tract is extremely painful and is often accompanied with diarrhea and vomiting. When HAE is not diagnosed, patients are sometimes thought to be imagining their abdominal pain while as many as a third of them undergo exploratory surgery to diagnose its source.

About half of all HAE patients experience at least one episode of laryngeal edema. If untreated this can be fatal, perhaps in as many as 30-40% of cases. Laryngeal edema has been estimated to occur in about 1% of all HAE episodes.

Swelling of the urinary systems may leave patients unable to urinate. Other organs from the brain to sexual organs are affected.

Patients experience episodes every other week on average with some patients having maybe one or two episodes a year, while others have them every few days. Attacks usually last three to five days but some are much longer. They generally develop more slowly than the allergic angioedemas, taking most of a day to fully develop. While most HAE is inherited, severity differs for each patient even within the same family.

HAE cause and triggers

The genetic defect causing HAE results in either low levels or defective blood proteins called C1-Inhibitor. C1-Inhibitor regulates inflammatory responses, coagulation, and infection control; without it, the peptide bradykinin builds up in the blood vessels and causes them to leak fluids.

There were originally two HAE types, both a result of mutations of chromosome 11:
- HAE Type I   The C1-Inhabitor levels are low
- HAE Type II   The C1-Inhibitor levels are normal but dysfunctional
- HAE Type III This type was discovered later and is very rare. The C1-inhibitor levels are normal. Type III involves an entirely different chromosome (chromosome 5). Most Type III patients are women, and the genetic mutation is inherited X-linked dominance. The clinical picture is different in that the onset is later, and there are fewer episodes. Type III sufferers also often suffer from swelling of the tongue, which can cause fatal asphyxias. The C1-inhibitor levels are normal except they fall when estrogen levels are high as in pregnancy and hormonal contraception.

Trauma is the most common trigger for HAE. It doesn't have to be an automobile accident kind of trauma. Sometimes just putting weight on one foot for too long can trigger an episode, or pushing something heavy, gardening and housekeeping. Dental procedures are also an important trigger, with symptoms appearing within six hours.

Stress and anxiety are the next most common trigger. When William Osler described HAE in 1888 he named it angio-neurotic angioedema. The 'neurotic' part of the name is understandable. Stress and anxiety are triggers and also symptoms of this condition: once a patient experiences a serious episode and knows it will happen again, it's hard for them to not become stressed and anxious.

Other triggers include:

- Menstruation, pregnancy, oral contraceptives, hormone replacement therapy
- Surgery
- ACE inhibitors for high blood pressure

Diagnosis

The diagnosis of HAE depends primarily upon taking patient and family histories and assessing the result of blood tests for C1-Inhibitor. Some less expensive tests may be run first, usually antigenic C1, C4, and C4 levels as HAE patients usually have low C4 but normal C1 and C3 levels.

Treatment

The drugs used for other types of angioedema are ineffective for the inherited types. These drugs include epinephrine, antihistamines, and corticosteroids.

The earliest effective preventive treatments for HAE were attenuated androgens (anabolic steroids); this includes drugs such as Danazol and Stanozolol. Attenuated androgens have been prescribed since the 1970s and are still used by many patients. They are given as a daily oral medication to reduce the frequency and severity of episodes; in half of patients episodes are completely, or nearly completely, prevented. The drugs are not without side effects: weight gain, hypertension, menstrual disturbances, virilization, increased serum lipid levels and liver toxicity occur in some patients. Liver studies before and during treatment need to be performed and their use in pregnancy and breast-feeding avoided. Generally these drugs are not given to children.

Until the late 1970s, there were no effective treatments for a severe attack, although some patients have benefitted from taking extra amounts of their anabolic steroids. Fresh, frozen plasma has been tried but has drawbacks.

In Europe in the late 1970s, effective drugs were developed to stop the acute attacks by using purified C1-inhibitor from human blood. These drugs were not approved by the FDA until the mid-2000s. Since then, research has continued to add to drugs that are available as treatment of acute attacks or as a preventive. The lives of patients have been improved by the move from hospital or office-based care to the training of patients to administer the drugs themselves.

Brand names of HAE drugs now licensed in the US and UK are listed below. Most can be given to adults and adolescents. All but Cinryze are given to allay an acute attack. The human C1-Inhibitors, Cinryze and Berinert are being used to treat children.

Cinryze (manufactured by ViroPharma)

Cinryze is a C1-Inhibitor concentrate purified from human blood. It is used to prevent HAE attacks of patients having frequent and serious attacks. It is delivered intravenously twice a week and is approved for home infusion. There is a rare risk of anaphylaxis so epinephrine must be available at time of infusion.

Ruconest (manufactured by Salix)

Rhuconest is a recombinant C1-Inhibitor that is purified from the milk of female rabbits that are genetically altered to produce the human C1-Inhibitor protein. Rhuconest is given by slow intravenous injection. Rhuconest is not a blood product and can't be given to patients with a rabbit allergy. Patients can inject the drug themselves.

Berinert (manufactured by CSL Behring)

Berinert is a concentrate of C1-Inhibitor. It raises the level of C1-Inhibitor in the blood and halts the progress of an acute attack of edema. Berinert is purified from donated blood plasma. Berinert has been used extensively over three decades and has an excellent safety record. The drug is FDA-approved for treating acute attacks and is delivered intravenously. It has approval for patient administration. There is a rare risk of anaphylaxis so epinephrine must be available at time of infusion.

Firazyr (Manufactured by Shire)

Firazyr is a synthetic protein and it is effective in halting an attack of edema by attacking bradykinin. Firazyr is given by subcutaneous injection. Some patients experience pain at the injection site. Patients can administer the drug themselves.

Kalbitor (Manufactured by Dyax Corp)

Kalbitor inhibits the inflammatory process in the tissues. It can therefore halt the progression of an attack of HAE. Kalbitor is given by subcutaneous injection. This drug must be administered by a healthcare professional.

Prevention

Dental treatments and surgery are the only situations for which drugs may be given prophylactically to prevent attacks. In those instances, one of the purified C1-Inhibitors is often prescribed. Before these drugs were available the anabolic steroids were given several days before and after a procedure; this is still the practice, especially if the drugs are known to be effective for the particular patient.

Patients are counseled to avoid physical trauma as much as possible.

Prevention of serious airway obstruction includes knowing the symptoms of an attack. In HAE the attack may develop over several hours but the medications used to stop them are most effective when given early on. If the attack starts deep in the throat, the throat may be itchy or sore and then progress to feeling something is lodged in the throat. The voice may get squeaky, higher pitched or the patient may have a barky cough. The patient then may have difficulty breathing. The attack may start instead with swelling of the lips and tongue and then spread towards the throat.

Patients are taught to carry a notice with them to notify any healthcare professional that the patient is NOT suffering from an allergic attack and requires specific medication. When travelling patients take medicines needed for an acute attack with them. Patients are also warned to seek medical care after treating themselves for an acute attack. Sometimes the medicines are not entirely effective and additional doses are needed.

The orphan drug world

There are only an estimated 6,500 to 10,000 people in the US who have HAE, and not all of them will need the newer medications. To develop any drug is expensive and to develop a drug for such a small population in need means the expense is shared by fewer people. So after the good news that medicines have been developed for HAE comes the bad news: the drugs are among the most expensive.

In the US, a year's treatment of Cinryze when given at the recommended two infusions a week cost $540,000 to $590,000 (£362,000-395,000) per year based upon pharmacy list prices in the US. The new treatments for acute attacks cost $6,000 to $10,000 (£4,000-6,700) per attack – and could potentially be double that if the first dose of the drug is not effective.

Who pays that much?

The drugs are covered in the US and UK as necessary by governmental and other insurers. There are, of course, some barriers:

In the US, insurers will require written diagnostic proof. Some want letters from an allergist or immunologist. Some will want proof that the tests necessary to diagnose the condition have been done. Some will state the minimal number of attacks per month and prior laryngeal attacks before paying for the newer drugs. Others require that the patient has tried anabolic steroids without success or have conditions such as liver disease that prevent them from taking the androgen. Some allow prescriptions for a single syringe of a drug to stop an acute attack when two doses may be needed.

When the medicines are covered by insurance plans they restrict the number of doses and place them in tiers that require high copays; often 33% or higher.

Most of the drug manufacturers offer programs to help some patients pay for the drugs. Some offer a free sample for physicians to use for a new patient.

In the UK, the necessary drugs are part of the NHS but there are still barriers to care. One probable sufferer of HAE wrote that her physician wouldn't order the needed tests for C1-Complement as once she had the diagnosis the costs would affect the health trust he worked for. This issue has also occurred in the UK in prescribing diagnostic scans for cancer.

Other barriers to care

A huge barrier to effective care of HAE is the delay in its diagnosis. It's a rare disease with symptoms occurring sporadically, especially at first. The symptoms also are short lived – they either go away in a few days each time or the patient dies from laryngeal swelling. Studies have shown at least a 9-10 year delay from when the patient has first shown symptoms to the HAE diagnosis.

Support and Information Organizations

There are a number of organizations that provide good information about HAE and provide other services to patients and their families as well as physicians caring for them. For example:

www.haehope.com
This is a site sponsored by Dyax, manufacturer of Kalbitor. Dyax offers a program to refund copays of genetic testing of patients not covered by government health programs by states or the US government.
Membership is free; benefits include a newsletter and access to experts.

www.angioedema.net
This site offers good, simple explanations of angioedema written by non-professionals and a reference list of medical literature. Not a membership site.

www.haea.org
Membership includes patients, families, and caregivers.
Membership is free.
The haea provides patient service teams that provide physician referrals, disease education, and individualized patient support. There is an emergency phone number on the site for the teams.
Has Facebook pages for adults and teens.
Advocacy group; standard setting group; provides CME courses

www.haei.org
International HAE organization.
Has good basic information plus world map to see which drugs are licensed in which countries and where HAE organized care groups are.

www.haeuk.org
Basic information.
Offers patient support in arranging for diagnosis and care
Supports an annual conference for patients and healthcare providers

www.patient.co.uk
This is a website for diseases in the UK written by physicians and includes a good discussion of HAE
There is also a patient leaflet available for HAE.
There is a section for asking advice about diagnosis or treatment of HAE.

Facebook:

Hereditary angioedema
This closed group 1100+ members with several subgroups. It has 5 administrators

Hereditary Angioedema (HAE)
Community closed groups for adults and teens for members of US HAEA only
Neither physicians nor representatives of pharmaceutical companies, research firms, marketing companies, or investment firms are allowed to join the Facebook groups

B. Anaphylaxis

Anaphylaxis is a medical emergency caused by an allergic or hypersensitivity reaction, which can be life threatening or fatal when the circulatory system suddenly leaks as much as half its fluid. There is no laboratory test for it; the diagnosis is made based upon the patient's symptoms and the medical history if it is known. It is often defined as two or more of the following symptoms occurring rapidly after exposure to the likely trigger: involvement of skin and/or mucosa, signs of respiratory compromise, falling blood pressure or end-organ dysfunction, and persistent gastrointestinal symptoms (end organs are major organs fed by the circulatory systems and include the heart, brain, eyes, lungs, and kidneys).

Symptoms

Severe symptoms can appear within minutes of the trigger – usually an allergen – and usually reach their maximum within 3-30 minutes. Occasionally other reactions follow hours later. Common symptoms of an attack are shown below.

- A sense of doom
- Itching and/or swelling of the mouth and throat. May be difficult to breathe
- Itching and/or swelling of the skin with redness, hives, or angioedema.
- Itchy watery or bloodshot eyes
- Increase in heart rate (which can change to low heart rate if loss of fluid from circulation is extreme)
- Nausea, vomiting, diarrhea, cramps,
- Weakness, confusion, fainting, loss of consciousness
- Incontinence

As anaphylaxis is diagnosed primarily by its symptoms. Grades of severity are used in many medical specialties to help decide when "watch and wait" is called for and when definite treatment should be provided, but it always comes down to clinical judgment. Early stages of anaphylaxis are similar to those of angioedema. Later stages show more organs involved and the severity of symptoms increase (appendix A contains a list of symptoms in a four-level grading system).

Mechanism of Anaphylaxis

Anaphylaxis is the body's reaction to chemicals released by mast cells and basophils, both white blood cells made in the bone marrow. Mast cells mature and live in connective and mucosal tissues while basophils circulate in the blood. When activated, they both release granules. Many of the granules contain chemicals like as histamine, which are called anaphylaxis mediators. When these substances are released, other inflammatory cells also become involved.

These anaphylaxis mediators can cause *extreme* vascular leaking: within ten minutes as much as 30-50% of vascular volume can flood the extravascular spaces. This is the root cause of low blood pressure, fainting, irregular heart rate, or heart attack, which are symptoms of severe anaphylaxis (when bodies of those who die from anaphylaxis are examined, the heart often contains no fluid at all from its escape out of the circulatory system).

The anaphylaxis mediators also cause muscle spasms and increase mucous secretion of the respiratory and gastrointestinal systems. For the respiratory system, this leads to swelling of the throat and nasal passages, a cough and shortness of breath. Gastrointestinal symptoms include difficulty swallowing, nausea, vomiting, diarrhea, bloating, cramps and pain.

There are books written about the cascade of anaphylaxis mediators and their effects on the body. These details are beyond the scope of this chapter. But given the location of the mast cells and basophils throughout the body almost every organ can be affected – if not at first, following the drop in circulation.

In adults, symptoms usually occur first in the skin and mucous membranes (hives, rash, or angioedema) followed by respiratory, circulatory, and gastrointestinal systems. Children, however, usually have respiratory symptoms first.

Who gets anaphylaxis?

The incidence and prevalence of anaphylaxis can only be estimated as different clinicians identify it differently. Some include only the most severe cases while others include early stages of the condition. Even deaths from anaphylaxis can only be estimated because of coding differences: in the US, estimates range from 500 to 1500 deaths a year. An estimated 0.03- 0.05% of the population has a severe attack once a year – that's 3 to 5 people per 10,000. Estimates of the lifetime risk for any person is 1-2%. A greater number of people are at risk of an attack but estimates of this population also differ greatly – ranging from 15-30%.

In the US, a random telephone survey of adults collected data for the prior ten years (Wood, 2013). That study concluded that 5.1 % of the sampled 1000+ adults probably had experienced anaphylaxis and that 1.6% very likely had experienced an attack. In that study the triggers were:

34% ... Medicines

31% ... Foods

20% ... Stings

15% ... Other, or no known trigger

Anaphylaxis can occur at any age, with age specific rates highest for those under 17 years old. Males have lower rates in most studies. Triggers vary by age with younger patients more likely to have food triggers.

There seems to be agreement that serious allergic anaphylaxis is increasing; these estimates are based upon following consistent data from small populations.

A major risk factor for anaphylaxis from many triggers is atopy, which is a genetic tendency to develop quick allergic reactions to substances in the natural environment. These substances include food, pollen, molds, mites, and dander. These patients include those with asthma, hay fever, and dermatitis. In studies about 40-50% of anaphylaxis attacks are of atopic patients. Atopy seems not to be a risk factor in penicillin allergies or insect stings.

Causes of anaphylaxis

Allergic reactions. Allergic reactions cause most cases of anaphylaxis. In allergies, the substance that causes the allergy is called an antigen. When an antigen comes into contact with the body, the body's immune system may protect itself by making antibodies. The particular type of antibody involved in allergic reactions is called immunoglobulin E (IgE). IgE is made the first time the body meets an antigen attaches to mast cells and basophils. There are no symptoms during this first meeting. The next time the body meets the allergen, however, the antigen binds to IgE already attached to the mast cells and basophils and causes them to release their granules, which contain histamine and other compounds, creating an allergic reaction that can involve the whole body.

Substances that can trigger anaphylaxis are many but most attacks are triggered by food, medicines, or insects. The cause of a small number of attacks remains unknown even after careful study of the patient and are labeled "idiopathic".

Foods. Foods known to cause anaphylaxis are the same as those causing allergic angioedema; mainly peanut, tree nuts, fish, shellfish, milk, eggs, seeds (such as sesame, psyllium, mustard), fruits and vegetables. Almost any food protein is capable of causing anaphylaxis.

If someone is allergic to a food product, occasionally anaphylaxis can happen just by breathing it. This can happen when the proteins are carried by steam in cooking or upon opening a package. In addition, if a person has a severe allergy to pollen, later anaphylaxis can occur when eating food that contains the same or similar protein. Persons allergic to ragweed, for example, may also react to melons and bananas; those with latex allergies may also react to several fruits, including bananas, papaya, and avocado.

Exercise plus food. These are strange allergies in which a person is not allergic to a particular food or to exercise, but exercise a few hours after eating a food causes anaphylaxis.

Medicines. Penicillin is the most common trigger of anaphylaxis. The attack is most serious when the drug is injected. The part of the chemical's structure that is responsible for the reaction is beta-lactam. Other antibiotics that contain beta lactam can also elicit anaphylaxis; many are listed in Appendix B.

Anesthesia. Various drugs used in anesthesia cause anaphylaxis. Perhaps the most common type of drug doing this is the neuromuscular blocking agent known as muscle relaxants. These agents cause direct release of histamine.

Insects. The enzymes in the venom of several insect species can cause anaphylaxis. These insects include bees, yellow-jackets, wasps, and fire ants.

Latex. Latex is a natural product made from the rubber tree. Latex is found in condoms, rubber gloves, toys and office products. The use of latex gloves in medicine, dentistry, and food service have caused allergies and sensitivities among staff and those they come into contact with. Powdered gloves are especially a problem as the cornstarch absorbs the latex protein and works itself more closely into the skin; also when the gloves are removed it puts the latex proteins into the air causing danger for those nearby who may be allergic.

Side effects of allergy treatment. Treatments to reduce serious allergic reaction include injecting small, then larger, amounts of the involved allergen over a long period of time. These treatments can result in anaphylaxis. This is why they are given in a medical setting and require the patient to wait up to an hour after the injection.

Proteins foreign to the patient. People can become allergic to fluids from another person, such as semen. Proteins used in medicine can cause anaphylaxis after repeated use: this has occurred with insulin treatments as well as the newer immunologic treatments for cancer.

Non-allergic reactions

There are some non-allergic causes of anaphylaxis. These act through other chemical routes to cause mast cells and/or basophils to release their granules.

Systemic mastocytosis is a cancerous condition in which mast cells multiply and infiltrate many organs of the body including bone marrow, skin, gastrointestinal tract, liver, and spleen. Patients are at risk of exaggerated reactions – including anaphylaxis – to food and insect venom and are warned to avoid substancex known to directly affect mast cells such as alcohol and opioids.

NSAIDs. Aspirin and other non-steroidal anti-inflammatory drugs such as Motrin, Advil, ibuprofen, and Aleve have caused anaphylaxis. Patients with known sensitivities to these medicines are warned to read the labels of medicines containing a mixture of drugs such as Midol.

Sulfites. Sulfites are thought to cause allergies and anaphylaxis through both allergic and non-allergic pathways. Sulfites are turned to gas in the stomach and then inhaled.

Sulfites were once added to fresh foods in grocery stores and restaurants to stop them from turning brown. Their link to serious reactions led the FDA to ban this use in 1986. The FDA also requires warning labels on any food containing more than 10 parts per million, an amount thought to be safe.

Foods with very high levels of sulfites include wines, beer, dehydrated or dried fruit (except for dark raisin and prunes), cut potatoes, shrimp, fruit jelly, foods containing dried fruit (trail mix, cereal, baked goods, etc.), syrup, maraschino cherries, soup, baked goods, canned and frozen fruits and vegetables, condiments, relish, fruit juice, seafood, packaged lemon or lime juice, soft drinks, tomato products, and parmesan cheese. (Appendix C lists foods and medicines that may contain high levels of sulfites).

The FDA regulates the ingredients for food products and prohibits products known to contain natural high sulfite levels.

Exercise. Exercise alone or with another trigger such as food or pollen can lead to anaphylaxis. Studies have shown that attacks become less frequent over time but reasons for this include the suspicion that many patients simply exercise less frequently or with less intensity.

Progesterone. Occasionally, a woman becomes hypersensitive to her own progesterone during menstrual cycles.

Blood and blood products. Anaphylaxis can occur when either whole blood or any of its components are given. Some unusual reactions are caused when patients missing a blood component altogether are given them as treatment – the body interprets the missing protein as a foreign body and reacts to it after repeated doses.

Contrast materials in radiology. Contrast materials that are injected for radiographic studies of the heart, urinary tract, etc. are often iodine-based. The original contrast material was painful for the patients and caused kidney damage; one study found that about 13% of the patients had an adverse reaction, with 0.20% of them severe. Contrast materials were modified and the newer low osmolar non-ionic material didn't cause pain on injection; all adverse reactions were reduced to 3% of patients, and severe/very severe reactions to 0.04% (Katayama, 1990).

Treatment

Once an attack has occurred, treatment is supportive and entails keeping the body functioning until the attack has subsided.

The first line of treatment is epinephrine, usually given intramuscularly in the mid outer thigh. Epinephrine is also known as adrenaline. It is a hormone secreted by the adrenal gland; for medical use it is a synthesized product. In anaphylaxis the drug tightens blood vessels, stopping the leaking and increasing blood pressure. It also relaxes the respiratory muscles making it easier to breathe. In about 25% of cases more than one epinephrine injection is required, given every five to fifteen minutes until the attack subsides; in serious attacks the drug may be given intravenously. Further treatments include antihistamines, IV fluids, bronchodilator, oxygen, and CPR.

Patients are monitored for some time to assure treatment for a possible second attack is adequate. Estimates of the frequency of later attacks vary all over the place, from 1-25%. Some are inherently biphasic but others result from inadequate treatment of the initial episode. These later attacks can occur as soon as an hour or be delayed for three days; most occur within 12 hours.

Patients are warned to call for emergency help after self-injecting adrenaline. At this point they may have lost much of their circulating fluid. While waiting, they are told to lie on their backs (and remain on their back) with their legs raised. Deaths have occurred when patients are raised to a standing or sitting position after a severe attack before they have received adequate fluid – this causes blood to pool in the lower extremities, stealing oxygen from the brain and heart.

Patient care issues

Access to epinephrine, especially in self-injectors. In an ideal world, patients at risk of anaphylaxis would be prescribed self-injectors prefilled with an appropriate dose of epinephrine to treat an impending attack early. The earlier the epinephrine is given, generally the better the outcome. A serious attack can result in a quick death, which prevents travelling to get epinephrine; patients can be having what seems like a normal allergic episode but within minutes other, serious symptoms arise. Some patients don't have access to epinephrine while others are prescribed syringes and vials of the drug. Filling a syringe while nervous or experiencing an attack is a barrier to care. In addition, patients may not carry the materials with them when they are away from home.

Unfortunately, a recent survey of adults in the US who have had an anaphylaxis attack found that while most had experienced two or more attacks, half had never received a prescription for epinephrine and 60% did not have any available at the time of the survey (Wood, 2013).

Data clearly show that anaphylaxis deaths occur more often when patients are away from home and are associated with either not using epinephrine or with a delay in the use of epinephrine. Other issues include not calling for emergency care after epinephrine was given. Occasionally in obese people with deep subcutaneous tissue, the auto-injectors don't reach the muscle with a full dose.

The CDC licenses each self-injector separately so patients will always have a familiar product; when getting refills patients are warned to be sure to receive the product prescribed.

Training kits with empty syringes are used for teaching kids and their family how to inject the drug. These training sessions need to be repeated frequently with assurances that it's better to use the drug than not.

On the research front, scientists are trying to make an effective oral form of epinephrine. Animal studies on rabbits (they don't react to epinephrine) have progressed using microcrystals of epinephrine in a tablet form, which disintegrates in seconds when placed under the tongue (Rawas-Qalaji, 2015).

Misdiagnosis. Misdiagnosis is also an issue as many patients already have asthma and pursue treatment for that instead of for anaphylaxis (Risenga, 2015). Many of the allergy associations provide good short diagnostic tips and directions for care to carry on the person and distribute to schools and places of work. (The World Allergy Organization has a searchable database of these associations). For parents, the CDC has a booklet *Voluntary Guidelines for Managing Food Allergies in Schools and Early Care and Education Program,s* which can be downloaded; it focuses on food allergies but many of the issues are transferrable to any allergy.

Prevention

Avoiding the allergen or trigger is the first and best line of prevention.

People at risk of anaphylaxis should wear a Medic-Alert bracelet that clearly states the trigger, the risk of anaphylaxis, and location of medications.

The allergist or immunologist may recommend a series of allergy shots for honeybee, hornet, wasp, yellow jacket or fire ant allergy. These shots are extremely effective (said to be 98% protective) for all but the fire ant. They may also treat food allergies by exposing patients to tiny but increasing amounts of the food. Anyone with a reaction to x-ray dyes is pretreated with a sequence of drugs, including steroids and antihistamines is a substitute dye is not feasible.

Research is ongoing to see if probiotics can play a helpful role in suppressing allergies and reduce the number of anaphylaxis attacks. This type of research is based upon the known link of "cleanliness" to allergies. Thus far World Allergy Organization has found a "likely benefit" of some probiotics in preventing eczema but based this on "very low quality evidence". (Fiocchi, 2015)

Another line of research in Sweden found babies had less asthma and eczema and were less apt to becoming sensitized to antigens in general when their mothers cleaned dropped pacifiers in their own mouths. The effect was thought useful by the transfer of useful bacteria from mother to child (Hesselmar, 2013).

Patient and family support

Many people who don't have family members with severe food allergies have no idea of the seriousness of the disease and the fear that kids and parents experience. Supportive websites are especially useful for this population.

A few of the many good websites to try:

Trigger
www.triggerallergy.com
This Australian site has two videos that are helpful in explaining food allergies to everyone. It also calls to light the meanness of people towards children with severe food allergies: adults and children alike making fun of them and even tricking them to eat the foods that can kill them. Trigger has a focus of educating entire communities about the danger of food allergies.

Food Allergy Research & Education (FARE)
www.foodallergy.org

The FARE website has a wealth of information that is well organized. Much of it is age-specific – teens, children, parents, etc. It provides explanations of proven tests for food allergies and why they work as well as tests that are not recommended. One of the sections has specific strategies for safety at home, at school, at the workplace, or when eating away from home or travelling.

FARE provides research grants, reports research results and information about open clinical trials.

Anaphylaxis Campaign
www.**anaphylaxis**.org.uk
The Anaphylaxis Campaign is a UK organization targeting those at risk of anaphylaxis. The organization has a YouTube channel with several videos, issues food alerts, and supports research. They've developed and sell access to three online educational programs called AllergyWise geared from the patient to physician. Nurses and physicians receive CME credits for the programs. There is a fee for membership, The Campaign has a large searchable information cache as well as a library of fact sheets about all the common allergens. Their help line is available by phone or email and is open to anyone.

Anaphylaxis Canada
www.**anaphylaxis**.org
Anaphylaxis Canada is a national organization focused on people at risk of severe allergic reactions. The site provides email alerts about food products and has comprehensive lists of types of food products that may contain a certain antigens. The information section is crisp and includes a section of key points for anyone dealing with someone caring for a person having an attack.

C. Hydrocephalus

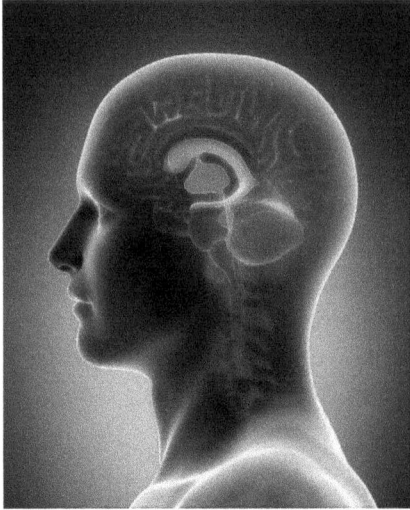

Picture: Cross-section showing normal brain ventricles

Hydrocephalus is defined primarily as having abnormally large ventricles of the brain. The brain has four ventricles that produce and hold cerebral spinal fluid (CSF). The two large lateral ventricles are in the cerebrum, the uppermost and largest part of the brain. The lateral ventricles are connected by narrow ducts to the third ventricle, which is lower, and in the midline of the brain, then another narrow duct connects the third to the tiny fourth ventricle. The fourth ventricle leads to the central spinal canal. In addition to large ventricles, the diagnosis of hydrocephalus includes an assumption that there is a defect in the flow, absorption, or production of CSF.

Purpose of CSF

CSF performs several functions for the brain. It circulates nutrients, removes waste, and acts as a shock absorber to adapt to changes in blood volume being pumped to the head and to protect brain cells against external physical bumps. CSF is 99% water and is normally crystal clear. CSF is made from serum in the blood through filtration and some active transport. CSF has many of the same concentrations of substances as serum except for protein – CSF has 35 mg/dL of protein while serum has 7000 (the brain makes its own protein).

Size of the brain ventricles

In normal brains the ventricles are small; in a healthy adult they may hold 1-2 ounces (20-40 mL) of CSF. The size of the ventricles in hydrocephalus depends upon the age of the patient and type of hydrocephalus.

The skull bones of infants and children under 2 years old are not yet completely fused; if ventricular pressure increases in children of this age, their ventricles enlarge and push to expand the skull – often without damaging the brain. Infant hydrocephalic ventricles can hold as much as a quart (1000 mL) of CSF when measured before treatment (a newborn's total brain volume averages 370 mL, growing to 960 mL at one year).

In older children and adults, the skull won't expand if the brain is pushing against it. The ventricles can expand only so much before damaging the brain itself; adult hydrocephalic ventricles measured before treatment may hold close to a pint (500 mL) of CSF.

Note: Children and adults with undiagnosed, untreated hydrocephalus can have ventricles much larger than this before dying from the condition.

Causes of hydrocephalus

Most cases of CSF are produced by choroid plexuses located within each ventricle. About 17 ounces (500-700 mL) of CSF is produced in the ventricles every day. A choroid plexus is a mesh of capillaries that filters plasma from the blood to obtain nutrients and create CSF; it also recirculates CSF in the ventricles to remove waste.

CSF usually flows out of the ventricles through to the subarachnoid spaces directly over the brain and spinal cord and then into the vascular circulation via the arachnoid membrane. In some areas, the lymphatics are also involved in draining CSF. When there is a serious obstruction of that flow, hydrocephalus can result. In rare instances, hydrocephalus can occur if a tumor of the choroid plexuses causes overproduction of CSF.

In the more common types of hydrocephalus in infants, flow of CSF is obstructed within the ventricles or at the arachnoid membrane. These types are often called non-communicating when the ventricles are blocked and communicating when they're not. The blockage can be from hemorrhage, infections, tumors, or congenital malformations. Genetic disorders can be a direct or contributing cause of hydrocephalus.

Less common types of hydrocephalus are ex-vacuo and normal pressure. These are the more common types of hydrocephalus in adults.

In ex-vacuo hydrocephalus, the brain shrinks after being injured by trauma, stroke, or in advanced age or Alzheimer's disease. As the brain shrinks, the subarachnoid and ventricular spaces expand to fill the void with additional CSF. This type is considered by many to not be hydrocephalus at all as there is really no problem with CSF flow or production.

In normal pressure hydrocephalus (NPH), there is a restriction of the CSF pathway, which occurs slowly over time. The ventricles enlarge to handle the excess CSF and the enlargement causes brain damage but abnormal ventricular pressure isn't found. In some cases the cause may be traced to head trauma, brain surgery, hemorrhage, infections or tumor – but the cause is usually not discovered. When the cause is unknown it's said to be idiopathic. In NPH, the pressure may actually be slightly higher than normal – just not as high as found in other types of hydrocephalus. NPH is thought to be a condition of chronically impaired reabsorption of CSF by the arachnoid membrane.

Whether CSF is blocked at the ventricle level or at the arachnoid membrane, CSF continues to be produced and CSF pressure increases as it tries to get out. This increases the size of the ventricles, may compress and damage the brain, and may cause cerebral edema. But in most cases, a steady state is reached with the CSF pressure abnormally high but no further brain damage occurring.

Symptoms

Symptoms vary depending upon the cause of the hydrocephalus and the age of the patient.

Newborns and infants: When the CSF is blocked but the head can expand, there may be no symptoms at first other than the head growing faster than normal. Later symptoms include poor feeding, vomiting, drowsiness, failure to thrive, eyes pointing down (called sun-setting eyes), and seizures.

Older children and adults: With an intact skull, the symptoms in older children and adults include those caused by high CSF pressure. Common symptoms include morning headache leading to nausea and vomiting, clumsiness, gait changes, trouble seeing, lethargy, decline in intelligence, and large head.

Older adults: Normal pressure hydrocephalus usually occurs in older adults, generally those over age 60. The ventricles increase slowly in size and the area of the brain that is affected are those that control the legs, bladder, and the "mind" – memory, reasoning, speaking. NPH is difficult to distinguish from many other conditions, including Alzheimer's disease. The patients may stand and walk with their legs further apart, act as if their legs are glued to the ground, and walk bent over and unsteady, shuffling. Bladder problems range from urgency or frequency to incontinence. The problems of the mind include short and/or long term memory loss, a flat affect – apathetic, inability to focus.

Is hydrocephalus common?

There are no really good estimates of the incidence and prevalence of hydrocephalus. Hydrocephalus appearing in infancy, excluding congenital conditions, is thought to occur in about 1-2 per 1000 births. Congenital conditions such as spina bifida/myelomeningocele may account for that much again. In the US this would mean at least 8000 new infant cases per year. Estimates for the prevalence of hydrocephalus among those aged 18 years and younger have been estimated 0.9 per 1000 population, or 74,000 in the US. One estimate is that 9,000 new cases of hydrocephalus are diagnosed each year in the US. Overall estimates of all people living in the US with hydrocephalus range up to a million (Hydrocephalus Association and National Hydrocephalus Foundation, 2015).

What overshadows the numbers is the uncertainty of the number of NPH patients whose hydrocephalus has not been diagnosed or treated. These estimates range from 300,000 to a million – most of whom are undiagnosed or diagnosed too late to be treated successfully.

Diagnosis

Diagnosis includes taking a good medical history and performing a full neurological exam. High CSF pressure causes the fontanels, or soft spots of babies' heads, to be firm and taut. In addition, when looking at a patient's eyes, a healthcare worker can see if the optic nerve is compressed – this is one way to rule out normal pressure hydrocephalus when evaluating an older person.

The diagnosis of hydrocephalus is generally confirmed by a radiographic study of some sort, usually CT or MRI of the skull of older infants and adults and ultrasound in newborns and younger infants. If CSF pressures are not terribly high, these studies may be repeated over time to see if the hydrocephalus is static or resolving. Other studies may be performed as a guide for treatment to determine where a blockage to CSF may be occurring.

If a problem with a birth is suspected, ultrasound and even MRI can follow the fetus during pregnancy and a diagnosis be made before birth. Included in regular child health visits are measures of the head – these measurements are a useful alert to the need to consider hydrocephalus in young children.

In NPH, often CSF is removed and the patient observed to see if symptoms are alleviated before progressing to a permanent treatment.

Treatment

Shunts. The most frequent treatment of hydrocephalus is inserting a plastic shunt between the ventricles and elsewhere in the body – usually the peritoneal cavity. Shunting excess ventricular fluid to the outside was attempted as early as the 10th century with the first sterile ventricular drainage performed in the 1880s. The technology of modern shunts has improved over the years to include the ability to change the flow rate to avoid both overly high CSF pressure and taking too much fluid out and collapsing the ventricles – called slit ventricles. Plastics imbedded with antibiotic have been shown to reduce infections; one of the causes of needed shunt revisions.

Despite improvements, shunts are still a problem: many shunts fail and revisions or replacements are needed. Shunt failures have many causes: infections, clogging, breaks and disconnects, and the need for a larger size. Sometimes only a piece of the shunt needs replacing. The average life of a functioning shunt is thought to be about 6-10 years. Estimates are that a third of the shunts in children failed in the first year, and failure rate was 4.5% per year after that. A long-term follow-up study of pediatric patients showed the need for shunt revision (most of them total replacement) was for 85% of them over 15 years. (Stone, 2013)

In the US, of the estimated 40,000 shunt procedures performed each year only about a third are for the patient's first shunt.

Many infants are born with a history of ventricular hemorrhage, a common risk for hydrocephalus. These infants are monitored carefully. If CSF high pressure is indicated, a temporary reservoir is placed, with a tube going from the ventricle to a small reservoir under the skin of the head (these are called subgaleal shunts). Fluid is removed as needed to avoid high CSF pressure and enlarged ventricles. Many of these children later require permanent shunts but shunts in early infancy are avoided, as they are apt to fail because of the higher protein and multiple cells in infant CSF.

Fetal shunts make sense in that much brain tissue is lost as hydrocephalus develops before the baby is born. Inserting shunts into the heads of fetuses, draining the CSF into the uterus, has been tried successfully but the high complication rate has discouraged its continuation in the US. The biggest roadblock to success is being able diagnose the specific cause of hydrocephalus of a fetus, as only shunting for fetal ventricular duct blockage has been successful. Shunting has been performed both in a closed uterus using and in an open uterus.

Fetal surgery is already reducing the need for some shunts. Myelomeningocele is a congenital condition in which the backbone doesn't completely cover the spinal cord, leaving a protruding cord, usually in the lower back. CSF leakage often occurs, pulling the brain downwards in the skull, causing the blockage of the ventricles. When allowed to develop until term, almost all of these babies will receive a shunt at some time in their lives and account for at least 20% of all infant shunts. Surgery performed early in the pregnancy (19-26 weeks) to close the spinal cord has reduced the need for shunts in this population by about 40%.

Ventriculostomy. Endoscopic third ventriculostomy (ETV) is becoming a standard treatment for hydrocephalus caused by obstruction of the ventricles. It is a surgical procedure that punctures the floor of the third ventricle, allowing CSF to drain into a subarachnoid cistern. This procedure was performed in the 1920s but then done infrequently with the advent of the shunts in the 1960s. Its resurgence has been the result of disappointment with shunt failures and improved endoscopic tools. Patient selection is critical for success of this procedure. Data comparing ETV with shunts show comparable patient outcomes (reduced ventricular size, lowered CSF pressure) while ETV has shorter operating room time, fewer post-operative complications and lower reoperation rates (Cheng, 2015). Sudden deaths have been reported when the opening made by the ETV closes.

Other operative procedures are being evaluated for hydrocephalus including coagulating the choroid plexus at the same time as ETV to lower CSF production and physically creating new openings in obstructed ventricular ducts.

Outcomes

Outcome data are muddied somewhat by the various populations and causes of hydrocephalus. A literature review of patients treated with shunts in the first year of life reflects a wide range of outcomes, which probably reflects a difference in the patient populations; the study found a mortality rates 0-3% from the disease and treatments; school difficulty 20-60%; cognitive problems 12-50%; and epilepsy 6-30% (Vinchon, 2012).

A German study tracked the results of children under a year old when treated with a shunt between 1971 and 1987. The group had reached an average age of 32 years old. The adults were 10% shunt independent; 40% had attended regular schools; 75% worked; 45% were independent; 35% depended upon their parents; and 20% were in institutions of various kinds (Preuss, 2015).

A study in Norway followed all children who had had their first shunt when younger than 15 years old. All were followed for twenty years. By then, 22% had died. Of the survivors, 56% were employed or in school, 23% worked in sheltered jobs, and 21% were unemployed (Paulsen, 2010).

A concern mentioned in both of the studies above was the difficulty of transitioning from child to adult, especially of a growing population depending upon aging parents, but also the need for follow-up care from pediatric specialists to adult physicians.

Prevention

Prevention of hydrocephalus involves preventing its causes.

Prenatal vitamins, specifically folic acid, a form of Vitamin B, lowers the risk of neural tube defects such as spina bifida/myelomeningocele, most of whom require shunts for hydrocephalus. The US government now requires certain foods to be fortified with folic acid; these foods include flour and products made from them. The rate of neural tube defects fell 30% in the ten years after passage of this law. In nature, folic acid is high in many vegetables and fruits.

A common cause of hydrocephalus of the newborn is ventricular hemorrhage, which is most prevalent in **premature births**, especially those born ten weeks before full term. Prevention of premature births is possible by taking folic acid a year before becoming pregnant and during pregnancy; avoiding smoking, alcohol, and illegal drugs; and reducing obesity. So far, premature births have not decreased in the US, increasing slightly overall, although the rate of very preterm births (less than 32 weeks' gestation) has not increased from 1990 to 2013.

Head trauma of all ages is another preventable cause of hydrocephalus. In the US, hospital use from traumatic brain injury (TBI) per 100,000 people increased from 2001 to 2010: emergency room visits from 421 to 816; hospitalizations from 83 to 92; but deaths fell from 19 to 17. With the aging population, falls are the most common cause, followed by motor vehicle accidents, blunt trauma, and assaults. In the last 20 years there has been no appreciable reduction in TBI or its outcomes. Sports-related brain injuries to children and adolescents increased 60% from 1980 to 2011. Head trauma prevention is dependent upon avoidance of alcohol and driving anything from car to skate board, wearing seat belts, wearing a helmet in contact sports, biking, motorcycling, skate boarding, etc. TBI of children can be prevented by using car seats, and safe highchairs, swings, and strollers, and using gated stairways (Center for Disease Control and Prevention, 2013).

Preventing **infections** of the fetus and newborn is another critical area where prevention can avoid hydrocephalus. Many infections have been implicated in causing hydrocephalus, including mumps, bacterial meningitis, flu, HIV, and parasites. The more well known parasite of concern in the US is toxoplasmosis but another, eggs of a pork tapeworm, Taenia solium, is a growing concern within immigrant populations causing a disease called neurocysticercosis. Women of childbearing age do well to keep their immunizations current and these immunizations are reviewed and updated in early pregnancy.

Pregnant women should avoid being around sick people as much as possible and receive prompt treatment of any disease. Toxoplasmosis is frequently found in cats and rodents (hamsters, rats, mice). Pregnant women are warned not to handle kitty litter, to cook all meat and vegetables thoroughly, and to keep an extra clean kitchen.

Patient and Family Support

Many organizations provide information and support for hydrocephalus patients and families. A few are listed below. The major ones provide links to others.

Hydrocephalus Association
http://www.hydroassoc.org

HA is a US advocacy organization, raises money for research and physician training, and provides scholarships to students with hydrocephalus. This national organization has professional members ($250/£170 fee) and has support groups with closed Facebook pages in thirty states plus Nigeria. Any individuals can contact HA via hot line and email. HA has added 'cure' to its goals and supports basic and clinical research. There is well organized information on the site ... not just about the disease and its treatment but booklets and excellent practical sheets such as how to deal with multiple specialist physicians, how to ask for a second opinion and what information to gather beforehand, and navigating workplace and school issues. The information targets teens, young adults, parents, caregivers, and NPH issues. The HA offers frequent 'webinars' (Internet meetings covering a wide range of information targeted at different groups including scientific discussions of recent research). The webinars can be attended on line by simply signing up and allow questions from attendees. The webinars are stored in a library accessible to anyone. The organization coordinates with other research groups and has recently started a genetic database.

National Hydrocephalous Organization
http://www.nhfonline.org

The NHO is a membership organization ($40/£27 per year). The website has good information about hydrocephalus. Members have access to a hotline as well as help finding care or contact with other parents or adult patients. They help establish support groups and publish several brochures.

Spina Bifida & Hydrocephalus Association of Canada
http://www.sbhao.on.ca

This is a membership organization ($20-30/£13-20 per year) – but can check box if unable to afford - that supports patients and families through educational materials and referrals. Good basic information on the website. Has free information packets and also a free lending library of videos and books. Has an extensive list of resources available from community and government and works with the patients and families to get the help they need. Also sells other information. Provides some scholarships.

Shine (spina bifida, hydrocephalus, information, networking, equality)
http://www.shinecharity.org.uk

This UK organization provides information and support for patients and families. They work to with members (membership is free) to coordinate care with the National Health Service. They provide in-person, Internet, and telephone contact and address physical, mental, employment, and independent living. The website has basic medical information as well as detailed information about the various welfare financial issues.

D. Pleural Effusion

The pleura are thin membranes that wrap the outside of our lungs with two thin layers of tissue containing between them a bit of liquid that protects and cushions the lungs. The inner layer (visceral pleura) wraps around each lung and is stuck so tightly to the lung that it cannot be peeled off. The outer layer (parietal pleura) lines the inside of the chest wall. The very thin space between the layers is called the pleural cavity. A liquid, called pleural fluid, lubricates the pleural cavity so that the two layers of pleural tissue can slide against each other.

Normally there is just a tiny amount of fluid between the pleural layers – 2 to 4 teaspoons in each lung. This is enough to allow the lungs to expand and contract when we breathe. When there is too much fluid in the pleural cavity it's called a pleural effusion. The effusion is affected by gravity so fills up the bottom of the pleural space first.

How much is too much pleural fluid?

How much is too much depends on what kind of fluid it is, what caused it, and if the fluid is causing symptoms. While the pleural space has little fluid in it, every day the membranes produce much more – about 17 ounces a day. Usually no symptoms are felt until one of the lungs has about 10 ounces of fluid in the pleural space. A large effusion can have 90 ounces or more surrounding one lung.

Are both lungs always affected?

Sometimes just one lung is affected, other times two. This can give the physician a clue as to its cause: for example, an effusion caused by congestive heart failure is usually bilateral while one caused by a pulmonary embolism usually affects one lung.

Symptoms of effusions

Usual symptoms of a pleural effusion include shortness of breath, chest pain, stomach distress, dry cough, and hiccups. Shortness of breath and rapid breathing are the result of the lungs being blocked from expanding normally so less oxygen is taken with each breath. Chest pain may be slight or a sharp stabbing pain and generally comes from inflammation of the pleura.

As noted above, about ten ounces of fluid is usually needed in the pleural space of a lung to cause symptoms. Effusions related to cancer, TB, and after major surgery may not cause symptoms.

How common is it?

Estimates are that 1.5 million people or more experience a diagnosed pulmonary effusion every year. The most frequent causes are congestive heart failure, pneumonias, and malignancies.

What causes the effusions?

Pleural fluid comes mostly from the lungs, filtered through the cells of the visceral membrane and from capillaries in the membrane. While some fluid is reabsorbed by capillaries in the pleura, most of the fluid is absorbed by the lymphatic system in the parietal membrane. The lymphatics also drain cells and cell debris; studies have shown that lymphatics are quite expansive and, if healthy and not blocked, can handle 30 or 40 times the normal amount of fluid produced daily.

Effusions result when too much fluid is produced or something blocks its absorption.

Too much fluid often comes from high blood pressure (such as from congestive heart failure), which increases filtration of fluid from the lungs into the pleural space. White blood cells fighting inflammation or infection of the pleura or cancer cells in the pleural space can secrete a large volume of fluid. Asbestosis can cause abnormal pleural membrane cells that overproduce fluid.

If there is excess abdominal fluid under high pressure, fluid can also flow into the plural space through gaps in the parietal membrane. This can happen during peritoneal dialysis or from ascites.

Other causes of excess fluid are conditions that lower the protein content of circulating blood, reducing the ability of capillaries to attract fluids. This happens in some liver and kidney diseases and in malnutrition.

Blockage of the lymphatics is a major cause of effusions. Blockage can be caused by cancer cells, infections, inflammation or trauma. In addition to blocking lymphatics, some say effusions are caused by effusions. Normal pleural fluid is a light yellow clear fluid; it's low in protein and usually contains just a few white blood cells. When there is inflammation, infection, cancer, or trauma of the pleura, the additional substances in the fluid attracts water from capillaries and pleural cells – adding to the problem.

Almost all patients have pleural effusions following coronary artery bypass surgery. Usually the effusions are small but perhaps as many as 10% of patients have larger effusions which need to be drained several times before healing occurs.

Drugs such as crack cocaine can cause pleural effusions. There are also many medicines that by themselves can cause pleural effusions. They cover a wide range of drug types and, as more drugs are developed, the fear is that this list will be forever expanding. Drugs that have been reported to cause effusions include several cardiovascular drugs, ergot based drugs for headache and for Parkinson's; chemotherapy agents; anticoagulants; follicle stimulating drugs and many more. There is a nice paper online by Charis Moschos MD of Athens Medical School, Haidari Greece, titled *Drug Related Pulmonary Diseases* that is undated but goes into this in great detail. The mechanism for the drug's effects are many: hypersensitivity of the pleura to the drug; direct toxicity or poisoning of the pleural cells; and chemical inflammation or irritation. Some drugs cause effusions of both the lung and heart linings.

Diagnosis

A patient's history, symptoms, and physical exam often provide enough information to raise a suspicion. On examination, the chest has a dull sound when thumped. When using a stethoscope, the breathing sounds are dull. If the patient has sharp chest pain, a scratching sound is heard – a signal that the two layers of the pleura are not moving normally and may be inflamed.

Radiology studies. The liquid effusion obstructs the view of the lung in a plain x-ray. A plain x-ray will also show an enlarged heart if CHF is present. Ultrasound can show small effusions and CT and MRI can point to underlying conditions.

Examination of the fluid. Tapping the effusion can provide relief of symptoms and also clues as to the cause. Clear, low protein effusions usually come from a process elsewhere in the body, such as an increase of fluid coming from the peritoneal cavity or from increase vascular pressure. Analysis of the cells directly or by culturing them can pinpoint cancers and infections.

A surgical biopsy of the pleura or lung may be needed in some cases. Direct viewing of the lung itself – bronchoscopy – may also be used in diagnosis.

Treatment of effusions

The main aim of treatment is focused upon treating the cause of the effusions. This includes antibiotics for infections and diuretics for congestive heart disease. If the cause is not known and/or the effusions are large, the effusions are drained to relieve the symptoms.

If the effusions persist after draining and treating the probable cause, irritants such as talc or doxycycline are sometimes placed in the pleural space, causing the two layers to adhere and stop producing pleural fluid. This irritant procedure is called pleurodesis and is usually painful.

Recovery can sometimes be slow, as time is needed for the pleural membranes to heal. It may take weeks or months for treatable effusions to heal.

Prevention of effusions

Many infectious diseases that affect the lungs and cause effusions can be prevented by adhering to recommended immunization schedules for pneumonia, flu, measles, whooping cough, and chicken pox. Seek prompt diagnosis and treatment of tuberculosis.

Risk of pulmonary effusions can be lessened by following general good health habits such as not smoking tobacco or crack cocaine.

E. Ascites

Ascites is defined as having an abnormal amount of fluid in the peritoneal (abdominal) cavity. In a healthy person, almost *any* fluid in the abdominal cavity is not normal. The cavity is lined by two membranes like the lung is ... one layer covering organs and the other covering the abdominal wall. The membranes produce a fluid that lubricates and allows movement; it also has anti-inflammatory properties. In men there is usually no fluid and in women it may fluctuate between none and a bit over a half an ounce (0-20 mL). In extreme ascites over 20 quarts (20 liters) may be present.

Symptoms

There may be no symptoms at all noticed by a patient and the ascites is discovered only during an exam. The increase in abdominal fluid may occur slowly or very fast. As the abdomen expands, this is often the only symptom that brings a patient to the doctor. As fluid increases, patients feel a heaviness and pressure in their midsection. Shortness of breath may occur if the pressure pushes up against the diaphragm, squeezing against the lungs. Later patients may have swelling in the hands and feet.

How many people get ascites?

Ascites is a symptom. There are no good statistics for the number of people affected. Most, perhaps 80%, of those diagnosed with ascites have cirrhosis as the underlying cause. Cancers account for 10%, and a long, long list of conditions are the reason for the remaining. There are also many cases that are not diagnosed.

For a sense of the numbers, those with cirrhosis are at high risk for ascites. In the US an estimated 400,000 people have cirrhosis and about 60% go on to be diagnosed with ascites.

How does the fluid get into the abdominal cavity?

One of the major ways abdominal fluid increases is that fluid gets squeezed out of the liver. About 75% of circulating blood goes through the liver. Nutrients, hormones, necessary cells and substances are delivered to the liver by the portal vein. If anything blocks the portal vein, its pressure increases. Portal vein pressure increase causes vascular pressure in the liver to increase, which pushes fluid out of the veins into the extracellular spaces and into the abdominal cavity. This situation is called **portal vein hypertension.**

What increases portal vein pressure?

The vein can be blocked by tumors, by lymphatic disease, or it may be narrowed from a congenital defect. The major blockages are caused by liver cirrhosis, and congestive heart failure. **Liver cirrhosis** is towards the final stage of liver disease in which scarring replaces much of the liver's cells. These scars begin to block circulation in the liver and finally begin to restrict flow from the portal vein.

Congestive heart failure increases venous pressure body wide, including that in the portal vein.

Other sources of peritoneal fluid in ascites come from **inflammation, infection, and cancer** both from the liver, other abdominal organs (pancreas, kidneys, adrenal glands, ovaries), and of the peritoneal membranes themselves. Infections include bacterial, fungal, TB, and HIV. Ascites is sometimes the first sign of ovarian cancer.

Once some fluid gets into the peritoneal fluid it can attract additional water from surrounding vessels, especially if the peritoneal fluid has high protein content (as when it comes from cancer and infections) or if the vascular fluid is low in protein (as in cirrhosis when the liver stops manufacturing albumin or in severe malnutrition).

What diseases are associated with cirrhosis?

At least 60% of cirrhosis is from direct damage from **alcohol**. The liver has the capacity to dismantle many toxins, including alcohol. But any long-term exposure to toxins can lead to the death of liver cells and scarring – and this is what happens in chronic long-term consumption of alcohol.

In the US, the second most common cause of cirrhosis is **chronic viral hepatitis**. In time, these diseases will become less common with immunization, available treatments, and increased surveillance of the medical blood supply.

Obstruction of the bile ducts is another common cause. The liver manufactures bile and delivers it to the intestines to digest food. Bile ducts can become obstructed with gallstones, infection, cancer, congenital defects, and genetic diseases such as cystic fibrosis. Bile acids build up in the liver and begin to destroy liver cells.

Genetic diseases, especially hemochromatosis, are another frequent cause of cirrhosis. This is an inherited disease leading to excessive iron absorption, which poisons the liver and other organs. Only about 10% of people who inherit the genes for this actually store excessive iron. The iron poisons the liver over many years. Often the disease isn't recognized until the person is between 30 and 40 years of age. Men are five times as likely to have the liver damage. Northern European heritage is associated with the gene. If diagnosed in a timely way, continued liver damage is prevented by bloodletting.

Another genetic syndrome leading to cirrhosis is **autoimmune hepatitis**. The patient's immune system attacks its own liver cells, causing scarring. This condition is more common in women who account for about 70% of cases.

Nonalcoholic fatty liver disease occurs frequently among the obese and those with diabetes. Metabolic syndrome, often a precursor to diabetes can be also a cause; these are people with three of the following: large waist, high blood triglycerides, high blood cholesterol, high blood pressure, and high blood sugar.

Other toxins besides alcohol can cause cirrhosis. These include some workplace toxins and medicines. The more common drug culprit is **Tylenol** (acetaminophen) in the US. Other names for the drug are paracetamol and APAP. The drug has many brand names. Using the drug beyond the packaged recommendation has led to acute and chronic liver disease.

Diagnosis of Ascites

Ascites is usually staged depending upon the amount of fluid. In one staging system, stages 1-2 have small, barely detectable volumes, stage 3 is an observable amount, and stage 4 is when the volume of fluid is so great the abdomen is tense.

Physicians can distinguish belly fat from large volume ascites by percussing the abdomen with the patient lying on the back then lying on the side. The way ascites fluid falls along the flank is also a sign. In addition, if belly fat is the cause, there is usually excess fat on the belly and along the sides and back. In ascites, the huge belly is more localized to the front. If belly fat can be grabbed in your hands, you can feel the abdominal wall beneath it.

Removing and examining some of the fluid can sometimes point to the root of the fluid. Often the albumin content of the ascites fluid is subtracted from the serum albumin level. A high value indicates portal hypertension – fluid has been squeezed out of the liver and albumin remains in circulation. Low values indicate something else is happening the abdomen. Fluid is studied for infection sources and other conditions.

Ultrasound is also a good way to see fairly small volumes of ascites fluid; less than 500 mL can be detected (Physical exams are usually sensitive to volumes in the neighborhood of 1500 mL). Other studies, CT and MRI, are used to detect the sources of the fluid.

Treatment of Ascites

Treatment of ascites involves diagnosing the source of the fluid and treating that. If a large volume of fluid is present it is drained, often several times, while the peritoneal membranes heal and fluid stops. The draining procedure is called paracentesis.

Dietary sodium is severely restricted to encourage fluid to be taken up in the circulation. Diuretics (water pills) are often given to reduce total body fluid reduction. For grade 2 and 3 ascites, therapeutic intermittent paracentesis may be prescribed. If the ascites is felt to be "intractable" a shunt is sometimes placed to drain peritoneal fluid back into a vein.

If portal vein hypertension is the cause of ascites, a TIPS procedure may be performed (TIPS = Transjugular intrahepatic portosystemic shunt). This is an interventional radiology procedure in which some of the blood (and pressure) from the portal vein entering the liver is shunted directly to a hepatic vein and returned to the heart.

Patients with longstanding cirrhosis and ascites have a poor prognosis. Often the only treatment is liver transplant.

Complications of Ascites

Bacterial peritonitis can occur spontaneously and can spread to damage organs throughout the body. Patients with chronic ascites are told to seek medical help immediately with symptoms of abdominal pain or fever. Long-term antibiotic treatment is often required to tame this infection.

Hernias, umbilical and in the groin, occur when ascites pressure increases. Surgery can have serious complications, including death, especially in patients with cirrhosis. If possible surgery is delayed and often avoided altogether if ascites volume is first reduced and the cause of the condition treated.

Complications of treatment include a small risk that an organ, especially the intestines, may be perforated in doing paracentesis and lead to infection.

Prevention of Ascites

Prevention of ascites involves preventing the underlying causes.

Alcohol. Avoiding long-term consumption of alcohol beyond that considered safe is the best way to avoid cirrhosis and its many complications. Safe amounts of alcohol are thought to be 1 or less standard drink a day for women and 2 for men. Children and adolescents have no safe amounts. Women are advised to drink less than men as they are generally smaller and, even when the same weight as men, have less body water to dilute the alcohol and reduce its toxic effects on the brain or other organs.
A standard drink is defined by the US CDC as 12 oz. of beer, 5 oz. wine, or 1.5 oz. liquor.

Obesity. Maintain a body weight at least below the obesity level; this would be to avoid having a BMI of 30 or higher. Overweight is considered between 25 and 29. BMI is a crude measure of body mass. Calculators are available online. The formulas for BMI are:
BMI = [weight in pounds / (height in inches x height in inches)] x 703
BMI = [weight in kilograms / (height in meters x height in meters)]

Avoiding high blood sugar levels. Normal blood sugar levels are now thought to be below 100 mg/dL. Sugar taxes the liver and the pancreas and is the cause of most types of diabetes, a risk of cirrhosis.

Read labels of any medicine, over the counter or prescribed. Follow any warning instructions about drinking alcohol while taking the medicine.

Medical care. In early liver disease, before it becomes scarred or fatty, the liver may become inflamed. At this stage there may be no symptoms as the liver enlarges. Regular medical physical exams and liver function blood tests can herald early liver disease. This is the time to seek definitive diagnosis and treatment. The liver has so many functions we cannot live without it: it manufactures proteins needed to carry oxygen, allow blood to clot, and allow the immune system to function; it stores and releases nutrients when we need them; it produces bile so we can digest food; it breaks down toxins; it breaks down saturated fats – just to name a few.

Patient/Family Support and Information Sources

There are three liver disease organizations that are very good places to receive direct support or information ranging from pamphlets to physician level video libraries. Non-liver causes of ascites such as heart and cancer diseases also have support organizations. Some small ascites chat spaces exist but seem to be unsupervised.

American Liver Foundation (ALF)
www.liverfoundation.org
This organization offers a packed website. Just a hint ... click on 'site map' at the bottom of the home page, that brings up the different topics at the top of the screen. Then when you click on a topic, say 'support', there is often a searchable feature related to the topic in the upper left corner.
There are no members. All features are open to all. ALF provides comprehensive information about liver disease, the many causes, drugs, research, and guides for new patients. The site also provides a comprehensive list of links to other organizations that may help.

There is a telephone helpline, links to ALF and other support groups in US and Canada, sources of financial support, discount drug card, written information, and online seminars.

Among the associated support services, ALF site provides directions to Caring Bridge. Caring Bridge supports free individual websites patients use to let friends and families know their progress. ALF also connects with Inspire – an international Internet site for sharing information.

Chronic Liver Disease Foundation
www.chronicliverdisease.org

This is an educational organization of liver specialists, a working group that has established educational centers throughout the US. Links to each site and photos of the liver specialists are provided. The organization reviews research and clinical practices, then provides educational resources to health care professionals treating patients with liver disease through the individual centers, large live meetings, and Internet meeting. The website has a searchable database of news articles, abstracts of medical literature, and videos/slide presentations from professional meetings. The site is organized by the initials shown below:

HBV – hepatitis B virus

HE – hepatitis encephalopathy, the brain's reaction to high ammonia levels resulting from poor liver function.

HCC – hepatocellular carcinoma, primary liver cancer

HCV – hepatitis C virus

NASH/NAFLD – NAFLD is non-alcoholic fatty liver disease; NASH is non-alcoholic steatohepatitis, a severe form of NAFLD

British Liver Trust
www.britishlivertrust.org

This organization provides a telephone help line, newsletter, educational meetings, and links to local support groups. Some of the support groups meet online, others have live meetings. There is a separate group for nurses.

A wide range of pamphlets are available for downloading, from explaining diseases and treatments to specific diets for different causes of liver disease. The site also has a good section explaining a wide range of diagnostic tests.

F. Anasarca

Anasarca is a term used to describe extreme generalized swelling of the skin over the whole body. The swelling is obvious.

By most definitions, the swelling involves only the subcutaneous layer of the skin. The subcutaneous layer is the bottom skin layer, below the epidermis and dermis. The subcutaneous layer contains mostly fat interspersed with large blood vessels, hair follicles, and sweat glands – held together with elastic fibers. This layer regulates body heat and cushions the body against injury.

While included in third-spacing conditions, anasarca's fluid isn't in a space between two membranes like the other conditions. Anasarca is often associated with other third spacing conditions, especially ascites and pleural effusions.

Anasarca is a symptom, not a disease. It usually signifies that the underlying disease has thrown fluid balance far out of control. The skin, being the largest organ of the body, offers a logical place to 'park' excess water.

Who is affected?

All ages from fetus to elderly.

Symptoms

Swelling occurs over a brief period of time; days or weeks. Swelling may have been noticeable in one part of the body first: extreme swelling above and below the eyes, marked swelling of the face, and swelling of the abdomen are common starting points. The swelling, when extreme, causes pain. An especially painful swelling may occur around the genitals, making urination difficult and painful for men. If the patient has stretch marks,

144

blister-like formations may poke through them, often leaking fluid. The patient's clothes may not fit. Hands and feet swell so they are hard to use.

Some patients experience dry, itchy, peeling skin.

The swelling of anasarca is a pitting edema; when you poke the skin with your finger it leaves a mark that is slow to bounce back. Pitting edema is the more common type of edema of the skin; it means that the lymphatics are functioning and can transport the displaced fluid. Only in myxedema and the later stages of lymphedema is there non-pitting edema (Myxedema is a very low thyroid condition. The skin swelling is in the dermis and composed of matter similar to mucous or joint fluid).

What causes anasarca?

The major causes of anasarca are usually having either too much sodium or too little protein in the blood.

- Excess sodium in the blood causes the body to retain water, increase blood pressure, and push water into extracellular spaces.

- Too little protein in the blood disrupts the fluid balance between capillaries and extracellular spaces. As there is more protein in the extracellular spaces it sucks fluid from circulating blood. Blood volume falls so the kidneys react by holding onto sodium, which causes the body to retain more water to leak into the extracellular space.

What causes the sodium increase that could trigger anasarca?
- Too much dietary sodium (rare)
- Congestive heart failure ... circulation to the kidney decreases, the kidney 'thinks' blood volume is the problems and retains sodium.
- Kidney failure where the kidney is unable to excrete sodium and it builds up in the body

145

What causes low protein that could trigger anasarca?

- Liver disease where liver reduces production of albumin
- Malnutrition: a general lack of protein in the diet
- Malnutrition: specific lack of an essential item in diet. For example, in babies transitioning from breast milk, iron deficiency anemia has resulted when babies fed cow's milk without iron supplements or when babies are fed 'healthy' milk such as rice milk, which has no protein and no iron. The anemia is thought to cause protein wasting through the gut.
- Kidney disease: nephrosis can cause the kidney to excrete protein
- Gastrointestinal disease especially those called protein-losing gastroenteropathies. Iron deficiency anemia was mentioned above. Other conditions include infections (bacterial, parasite, HIV), lymphoma, and Crohn's disease.

In addition to sodium and protein blood concentrations, other situations linked to anasarca include:

- Fetal/newborn conditions: About half of fetal/newborn anasarca is caused by the mother's immune response as it develops antibodies against fetal blood.
- Capillary leak syndrome: this rare condition, also known as Clarkson's Disease, affects middle-aged healthy people who suddenly develop recurrent attacks in which the capillary cells disconnect allowing proteins and fluids to escape. As much has 70% of plasma volume escapes to extracellular spaces within two or three days. This lowers blood pressure dramatically, and can cause multiple organ failure.
- Medicines: Medicines that can cause anasarca include corticosteroids and estrogens; some chemotherapy drugs such as docetaxel; calcium channel blockers for high blood pressure such as amlodipine; diabetes drugs in the

thiazolidinedione family; diazoxide used for both high blood pressure and diabetes; interleukin-2 immunotherapy for cancer, minoxidil used for both high blood pressure and promoting hair growth; NSAIDS (aspirin, acetaminophen, etc.).

- Autoimmune diseases, including juvenile dermatomyositis and autoimmune hepatitis
- POEMS syndrome is named for Polyneuropathy, Organomegaly, Endocrinopathy, Monoclonal gammopathy, Skin changes. POEMS is rare and associated with a disorder of bone marrow plasma cells which then affect other organs.
- Major surgery, especially of newborns and young infants
- Burns

How common is it?

As anasarca is a symptom of those seriously ill with a wide range of diseases, no good statistics are available.

Diagnosis

Diagnosis of fetal anasarca is done by ultrasound. The diagnosis is made when skin is thicker than 5mm (a US penny is 1.5 mm thick).

In newborns, fast weight gain is an indication of impending anasarca.

In children and adults, generalized thickening of the skin is evident on CT scans.

Patient history (including all medications), physical exams, electrocardiogram and laboratory tests are aimed at ferreting out the cause of anasarca. Tests of blood and urine for protein and electrolytes aid in the diagnosis of liver and kidney disease and protein deficiencies.

Treatment

Treatments aimed at the symptom of anasarca include diuretics to reduce fluid overload and albumin infusion in protein deficiency. The diseases that are the basic causes of anasarca all have varying protocols ranging from sodium avoidance in diet to transplanting liver or kidney.

Prevention

Fetal/neonatal anasarca

- Avoid infections. Numerous diseases can cause anasarca in the fetus or newborn. The list is long and includes parvovirus, CMV, syphilis, Coxsackie virus, rubella, toxoplasmosis, herpes, varicella, adenovirus, influenza, and listeria. A woman can't lock herself in a bubble but some precautions make sense:
    - Be current in immunizations.
    - If service is available, be tested for antibodies to fifth disease (parvovirus B19), a common infection often linked to anasarca. Having antibodies is a good thing.
    - Wash hands often
    - Don't rub eyes with hands
    - Avoid contact (hand shaking, kissing, sex) with obviously ill persons and limit contact with others
    - Avoid eating raw meat, unpasteurized milk
    - Practice safe sex/limit the number of partners
    - Avoid travel in high risk areas
    - Follow protocols for preventing Rh negative. Women with Rh negative partners to develop Rh antibodies that can attack the fetus's red blood cells.

- Thalassemia is a cause of many fetal deaths worldwide from anasarca. This is an inherited disease more common in Mediterranean countries and Southeast Asia.

Immigration trends lead many to forecast this disease to become more important in other countries, including the US. Estimates are that there are perhaps 1000 persons living in the US with the most severe form of thalassemia but no estimates of carriers are available. Preventing fetal deaths from this disease include finding carriers, pre-marriage counseling of couples, and early testing of the fetus. Often termination of the pregnancy is required although some have had success with fetal transfusions.

Infant anasarca

- Avoid profound iron deficiency anemia. When transitioning from breastfeeding, babies need formula with sufficient iron or supplements.

Children and Adults

- Prevention is primarily following a healthy diet, getting exercise, not smoking, drinking alcohol sensibly, avoiding illegal drugs, etc. – all to avoid heart, liver, and kidney diseases.
- Read the labels of prescription and over-the-counter medicines and follow instructions for dosing and for avoiding alcohol or other substances.
- Seek medical help early for sudden weight gain or puffiness

CONCLUSION

I hope that this book has taught you all that you need to know about water retention and, if not, has provided you with some useful links for further research. Please be aware that water retention is not always serious, however you should always seek medical attention just in case.

Thank you for reading this book.

APPENDIX

Appendix A

Grade of Severity of Anaphylaxis

GRADE I	GRADE II	GRADE III	GRADE IV
Skin	**Skin**	**Skin**	**Skin**
Erythema	Grade I signs	Grade I signs	Grade I signs
Angioedema			
Pruritis			
Urticaria			
Cardiovascular	**Cardiovascular**	**Cardiovascular**	**Cardiovascular**
No symptoms	Hypotension	Grade II signs plus:	Pulseless
	Tachycardia	Cardiovascular collapse	Cardiac arrest
	Presyncope	Profound hypotension	Death
		Bradycardia	
		Dysrhythmia	
Respiratory	**Respiratory**	**Respiratory**	
No symptoms	Dyspnea	Bronchospasm	
	Wheezing	Hypoxia	
Gastrointestinal	**Gastrointestinal**	**Gastrointestinal**	
No symptoms	Nausea	Grade II plus:	
	Vomiting	Incontinence	
	Diarrhea		
	Abdominal pain		
Neurologic	**Neurologic**	**Neurologic**	
No symptoms	No symptoms	Confused	
		Unconscious	

From: C. L Norred, A   Anesthetic-Induced Anaphylaxis, AANA Journal □ April 2012 □ Vol. 80, No. 2 page 133

Appendix B

Some antibacterial drugs containing beta-lactams

Penicillins Natural - derived from Penicillium sp. (Penicillin G or Benzyl penicillin)
- Penicillinase Stable (Resistant) Penicillins (Methicillin, Nafcillin)
- Isoxazolyl Penicillins (Oxacillin)
- Extended Spectrum Penicillins
- Aminopenicillins (Ampicillin, Amoxicillin)
- Carboxypenicillins (Carbenicillin, Ticarcillin)
- Ureidopenicillins (Azlocillin, Mezlocillin, Piperacillin)
- Beta-lactamase Inhibitor Combinations (BLI) (Ampicillin/sulbactam, Amoxicillin/clavulanic acid, Piperacillin/tazobactam, Ticarcillin/Clavulanate)
- Amidinopenicillin (Mecillinam)

Cephalosporins (Cephems)
- Cefazolin, Cephalothin, Cefamandole, Cefuroxime Cephamycin, Cefoxitin, Cefotetan, Cefmetazole, Cefotaxime, Ceftazidime, Ceftizoxime, Ceftriaxone, Cefepime, Ceftobiprole, Ceftaroline
- Oxacephem (Moxalactam)

Monobactams (Aztreonam)

Penems
- Carbapenems (Imipenem, Meropenem, Ertapenem)
- Penem (Faropenem)

Based upon: Customer Education Antibiotic Classification List, Vitek 2 Technology

Appendix C

Foods and medicines that may contain high levels of sulfites

FDA GUIDE TO FOODS AND DRUGS WITH SULFITES	
The following foods and drugs MAY contain sulfites, according to the Food and Drug Administration. Remember to check the product label.	
Food Category	**Type of Food**
Alcoholic Beverages	Beer, cocktail mixes, wine, and wine coolers
Baked Goods	Cookies, crackers, mixes with dried fruits or vegetables, pie crust, pizza crust, quiche crust, and flour tortillas
Beverage Bases	Dried citrus fruit, beverage mixes
Condiments and Relishes	Horseradish, onion and pickle relishes, pickles, olives, salad dressing mixes, and wine vinegar
Confections and Frostings	Brown, raw, powdered or white sugar derived from sugar beets
Modified Dairy Products	Filled milk (a specially prepared skim milk in which vegetable oils, rather than animal fats, are added to increase its fat content)
Drugs	Antiemetics (taken to prevent nausea), cardiovascular drugs, antibiotics, tranquilizers, intravenous muscle relaxants, analgesics (painkillers), anesthetics, steroids and nebulized bronchodilator solutions (used for treatment of asthma)
Fish and Shellfish	Canned clams; fresh, frozen, canned, or dried shrimp; frozen lobster; scallops; dried cod
Fresh Fruit and Vegetables	Sulfite use banned (except for fresh potatoes)
Gelatins, Puddings, and Fillings	Fruit fillings, flavored and unflavored gelatin, and pectin jelling agents
Grain Products and Pastas	Cornstarch, modified food starch, spinach pasta, gravies, hominy, breadings, batters, noodle/rice

	mixes
Jams and Jellies	Jams and jellies
Nuts and Nut Products	Shredded coconut
Plant Protein Products	Canned, bottled, or frozen fruit juices (including lemon, lime, grape, and apple); dried fruit; canned, bottled, or frozen dietetic fruit or fruit juices; maraschino cherries and glazed fruit
Processed Vegetables	Vegetable juice, canned vegetables (including potatoes), pickled vegetables (including sauerkraut), dried vegetables, instant mashed potatoes, frozen potatoes, potato salad
Snack Foods	Dried fruit snacks, trail mixes, filled crackers
Soups and Soup Mixes	Canned seafood soups, dried soup mixes
Sweet Sauces, Toppings	Corn syrup, maple syrup, fruit toppings, and high-fructose syrups such as corn syrup and pancake syrup
Tea	Instant tea, liquid tea concentrates

Source: University of Florida Document FCS8787, one of a series of the Family Youth and Community Sciences Department, UF/IFAS Extension.

REFERENCES

Agrawal V, et al. 2008 Dec. "Hyponatremia and Hypernatremia : Disorders of Water Balance." *japi* Vol 56 (ejournal).

Association for the Advancement of Wound Care. 2010. *Wound Care (AAWC) venous ulcer guideline.* Guideline, AAWC.

CDC. 2013. "CDC Grand Rounds: Reducing Severe Traumatic Brain Injury in the United States." *MMWR* 549-552 (Vol. 62 / No. 27).

Coney P, et al. Updated: Oct 6, 2014. "Menopause ." *Medscape Drugs & Diseases (online).*

Dash, P. ebook 2015 . "Blood Brain Barrier and Cerebral Metabolism." In *Neuroscience Online.* The UT Medical School at Houston.

European Society of Cardiolgy. 2013. ""Short-term smoking cessation reverses endothelial damage."."

Fareed, J. 2013. "Chronic venous disease (CVD): a condition of underestimated severity." *Current aspects in Chronic Venous Disease.* Rome: Alfa Wassermann/Springer Healthcare. 3-6.

Favero G, et al. 2014. "Endothelium and Its Alterations in Cardiovascular Diseases: Life Style Intervention." *BioMed Research International* Article ID 801896, 28 pages.

Ferré R, et al. 2012. "Effects of therapeutic lifestyle changes on peripheral artery tonometry in patients with abdominal obesity." *Nutrition, metabolism, and cardiovascular diseases: NMCD* 95-102.

Finnane, A. 2014. "PATIENT PERSPECTIVES OF THE IMPACT AND LONG - TERM MANAGEMENT OF LYMPHOEDEMA." PHD Thesis, Queensland University of Technology.

Fiocchi A, et al. 2015. "Guidelines for Allergic Disease Prevention." *World Allergy Organization Journal* Article 4, vol. 1, pages 1-13.

Flammer AJ, et al. Circulation. "The Assessment of Endothelial Function from Research Into Clinical Practice." *2012* 753-767.

Hesselmar, B, et al. 2013. "Pacifier Cleaning Practices and Risk of Allergy Development." *Pediatrics* e1829–e1837.

Kahn, S, at al. 2004. "Relationship between clinical classification of." *J Vasc Surg* 823-8.

Kapoor P, et al. 2010. "Idiopathic Systemic Capillary Leak Syndrome (Clarkson's Disease): The Mayo Clinic Experience." *Mayo Clin proc.* 905-912.

Katayama H, et al. 1990. " Adverse reactions to ionic and nonionic contrast media. A report from the Japanese Committee on the Safety of Contrast Media. ." *Radiology* 621-8.

Katz DL and Meller S. 2014. "Can We Say What Diet Is Best for Health?" *Annu. Rev. Public Health* 83–103.

Kimball, John W. n.d. "The Human Circulatory System: How It Works." Internet site: Kimball's Biology Pages.

Moore, Nicholas. 2015. *Renal Medicine.* e-report, www.fastbleep.com.

Nakamura, V. 2013. "A Patient with POEMS Syndrome: The Pathology of Glomerular Nephrotic Syndrom." *J. Exp. Med.* 229-234.

Onur, A. 2015. *Fluid Management.* e-report, www.fastbleep.com/biology-notes/15/31/205.

Paulsen AH, et al. 2010. "Twenty-year outcome in young adults with childhood hydrocephalus: assessment of surgical outcome,work participation, and health-related quality of life." *J Neurosurg Pediatr* 527–535.

Philips J, et al. 2012. "Characteristics, Mortality, and Outcome of Acquired Anasarca in the NICU." *e-Journal of Neonatology Research* Volume 2, Issue 3 126-129.

Plotnick GD, et al. 1997. "Effect of antioxidant vitamins on the transient impairment of endothelium-dependent brachial artery vasoactivity follow a single high-fat meal. ." *JAMA* 682-1686.

Preuss M, et al. 2015. "Adult long-term outcome of patients after congenital hydrocephalus shunt therapy." *Child's Nervous System* 49-56 (Issue 1).

Rawas-Qalaj M, et al. 2015. "Adrenaline (epinephrine) microcrystal sublingual tablet formulation: enhanced absorption in a preclinical model." *Journal of Pharmacy and Pharmacology* 20-25.

Risenga, M, et al. 2015. "Severe food allergy and anaphylaxis : treatment, risk assessment and risk reduction Severe food allergy and anaphylaxis : treatment, risk assessment and risk reduction : continuing medical education : continuing medical education." *South African Medical Journal* 72-73.

Rosenfeld, R, et al. 2008. "Hormonal and Volume Dysregulation in Women With Premenstrual Syndrome." *Hypertension* 1225-1230.

Rubinshtein R, et al. 2010. "Assessment of Endothelial Function by Noninvasive Peripheral Arterial Tonometry Predicts Late Cardiovascular Adverse Events." *EHJ* 1142-8.

Sachdeva, A, et al. 2009. "Lipid Levels in Patients Hospitalized with Coronary Artery Disease: An Analysis of 136,905 Hospitalizations." *American Heart Journal* 111-117.

Scallan, J, et al. 2010. *Capillary Fluid Exchange.* epublisher: Morgan & Claypool Life Sciences.

Schul, MW, et al. 2014. "Inequalities of health insurance guidelines for the treatment of symptomatic varicose veins." *Phlebology* 236-246.

Sinabulya H, et al. 2015. "Interobserver variability in the assessment of the clinical severity of superficial venous insufficiency." *Phlebology* 61–65.

Sovari, AA, et al. Updated: Oct 6, 2014. "Cardiogenic Pulmonary Edema." *Medscape REFERENCE* (online reference).

Stone J.J, et al. 2013. "Revision rate of pediatric ventriculoperitoneal shunts after 15 years." *J Neurosurg Pediatr.* 15-19.

Stranden, E. 2011. "Edema in venous insufficiency." *Phlebolymphology* Vol 18 (1): 3-14.

US FDA. Jan. 25, 2010. "FDA Approves First Percutaneous Heart Valve." U.S. Food and Drug Administration news release.

Vinchon M, et al. 2012. "Adult outcome of pediatric hydrocephalus." *Childs Nerv Syst* 847–854.

Vinchon M, et al. 2012. "Adult outcome of pediatric hydrocephalus." *Childs Nerv Syst* 847–854.

Weiss, R, et al. 2014 (online article, updated Oct. 1). "Venous Insufficiency." *Medscape Drugs & Diseases.*

wikibooks. 2015. *Human Physiology.* online book : wikibooks.

Wood RA, et al. 2014. " Anaphylaxis in America: The prevalence and characteristics of anaphylaxis in the United States." *J Allergy Clin Immunol.* 461-7.

Published by IMB Publishing 2015